Title

Unlocking Optimal Health: Embracing Our Ancestral Diet

Table of Content

Chapter 1

Introduction

In this introduction, we embark on a journey to explore the transformative power of ancestral eating. Throughout history, humans have adapted to diverse environments and diets, but it is the dietary patterns of our ancient ancestors that provide a compelling framework for understanding optimal nutrition. Ancestral eating emphasizes consuming whole, nutrient-dense foods that align with our evolutionary heritage, promoting not only physical health but also mental clarity and overall well-being.

To understand ancestral eating, we must first delve into the diets of our hunter-gatherer ancestors, who subsisted on a variety of wild plants, animals, and seasonal foods. Their diet was rich in protein, healthy fats, and fiber, providing essential nutrients for robust health and vitality. By examining archaeological evidence and studies of modern hunter-gatherer societies, we gain insight into the nutritional habits that sustained our ancestors for millennia.

Central to ancestral eating is the principle of nutrient density, which prioritizes foods that are rich in vitamins, minerals, and other essential nutrients. These include grass-fed meats, wild-caught fish, pastured eggs, organ meats, fruits, vegetables, nuts, and seeds. By focusing on nutrient-dense foods, we can optimize our nutritional intake and support optimal health.

Ancestral eating also emphasizes the importance of food quality and sourcing. Our ancestors consumed foods that were free from pesticides, hormones, and other harmful additives, instead opting for fresh, whole foods that were locally sourced and in season. By prioritizing organic, pasture-raised, and sustainably sourced foods, we can minimize our exposure to toxins and support environmental sustainability.

In addition to food choices, ancestral eating encompasses lifestyle practices that promote overall health and well-being. These include regular physical activity, adequate sleep, stress management, and social connections. By adopting a holistic approach to health that incorporates these lifestyle factors, we can enhance our resilience and vitality.

Throughout this book, we will explore the principles of ancestral eating in depth, examining the scientific evidence behind its efficacy and dispelling common misconceptions. We will provide practical tips and guidance for implementing ancestral eating in today's modern world, including meal planning, recipe ideas, and strategies for overcoming common challenges.

Ultimately, ancestral eating offers a powerful paradigm for achieving optimal health and well-being. By returning to the dietary and lifestyle habits of our ancestors, we can unlock the secrets to vitality, longevity, and resilience. Join us on this journey as we explore the transformative potential of ancestral eating and embark on a path towards greater health and vitality.

In this book, we will delve into the transformative power of ancestral eating, exploring its principles, benefits, and practical applications for optimal health. We'll begin by examining the evolutionary history of human nutrition and the dietary patterns of our ancestors. Then, we'll dive into the principles of ancestral eating, emphasizing nutrient density, food quality, and lifestyle practices that promote overall well-being. Throughout the book, we'll provide practical tips, guidance, and recipes to help you implement ancestral eating in your daily life. We'll also address common misconceptions and challenges, offering insights and strategies for success. Join us on this journey as we unlock the secrets to optimal health through ancestral eating.

In this comprehensive guide, we'll embark on a journey to explore the transformative power of ancestral eating, uncovering its principles, benefits, and practical applications for achieving optimal health and vitality. Throughout the book, we'll delve into the evolutionary history of human nutrition, examine the dietary patterns of our ancestors, and provide actionable insights to help you embrace ancestral eating in your daily life.

Our exploration begins with an examination of the evolutionary history of human nutrition. Throughout millennia of evolution, our ancestors adapted to diverse environments and diets, developing nutritional strategies that allowed them to thrive in their respective habitats. By studying the diets of hunter-gatherer societies and analyzing archaeological evidence, researchers have gained valuable insights into the dietary patterns that shaped human evolution.

Central to ancestral eating is the principle of nutrient density. Our ancestors consumed whole, nutrient-dense foods that provided essential vitamins, minerals, and other vital nutrients for optimal health. These included lean meats, wild-caught fish, fresh fruits, vegetables, nuts, and seeds, all of which were rich in micronutrients and bioactive compounds essential for supporting physiological functions and promoting overall well-being.

Ancestral eating also emphasizes the importance of food quality and sourcing. Our ancestors consumed foods that were free from pesticides, hormones, and other harmful additives, instead opting for fresh, locally sourced, and seasonal foods. By prioritizing organic, pasture-raised, and sustainably sourced foods, we can minimize our exposure to toxins and support environmental sustainability.

In addition to food choices, ancestral eating encompasses lifestyle practices that promote overall health and well-being. These include regular physical activity, adequate sleep, stress management, and social connections. By adopting a holistic approach to health that incorporates these lifestyle factors, we can enhance our resilience and vitality.

Throughout the book, we'll provide practical tips, guidance, and resources to help you implement ancestral eating in your daily life. We'll explore meal planning strategies, offer recipe ideas inspired by our ancestors, and provide guidance on sourcing quality ingredients. We'll also address common challenges and misconceptions surrounding ancestral eating, offering insights and strategies for success.

By embracing ancestral eating, you'll unlock the secrets to optimal health and vitality. You'll nourish your body with nutrient-dense foods, support your overall well-being with holistic lifestyle practices, and reconnect with your evolutionary heritage. Join us on this journey as we explore the transformative potential of ancestral eating and embark on a path towards greater health and vitality.

Chapter 2

The Evolution of Human Nutrition

The evolution of human nutrition is a fascinating journey that spans millions of years, reflecting the dynamic interplay between our ancestors and their environment. By examining the dietary patterns of our evolutionary predecessors, we can gain valuable insights into the nutritional strategies that shaped human physiology and behavior.

Our story begins millions of years ago, with the emergence of our earliest hominid ancestors. These early hominids, such as Australopithecus afarensis, inhabited East Africa and subsisted primarily on a diet of fruits, leaves, seeds, and other plant-based foods. Their diets were influenced by the availability of vegetation in their environment, as well as their anatomical adaptations for climbing and foraging.

As our ancestors evolved and migrated to new environments, their dietary patterns underwent significant changes. The emergence of Homo erectus approximately 1.9 million years ago marked a significant milestone in human evolution, as this species was the first to exhibit anatomical adaptations for long-distance running and hunting. With the ability to track and hunt game animals, Homo erectus expanded their dietary repertoire to include a greater proportion of animal-based foods, such as meat and marrow.

The transition to a diet rich in animal protein and fat had profound implications for human evolution. Animal foods are dense sources of essential nutrients, including protein, iron, zinc, and B vitamins, which are critical for supporting brain development, reproductive success, and overall health. The incorporation of animal foods into the diet provided our ancestors with a reliable and nutrient-dense source of energy, enabling them to thrive in diverse environments and adapt to changing climatic conditions.

The hunting and gathering lifestyle of our ancestors also played a key role in shaping their nutritional needs and dietary patterns. Hunter-gatherer societies typically exhibit a high degree of dietary diversity, consuming a wide range of plant and animal foods depending on the availability of resources in their environment. This dietary flexibility allowed our ancestors to adapt to a variety of ecological niches and survive in diverse habitats, from the savannas of Africa to the tundra of Siberia.

The advent of agriculture approximately 10,000 years ago marked a major shift in human dietary patterns. With the domestication of plants and animals, humans transitioned from a predominantly hunter-gatherer lifestyle to an agrarian society characterized by settled communities, crop cultivation, and animal husbandry. This agricultural revolution had profound implications for human nutrition, leading to changes in diet composition, nutrient intake, and overall health.

The shift towards agriculture brought about changes in the types of foods consumed, with an increased reliance on cereal grains, legumes, and domesticated animals. While agriculture provided a stable and abundant food supply, it also introduced dietary elements that were less prevalent in the ancestral diet, such as refined grains, sugars, and processed foods. These dietary shifts have been linked to an increased risk of chronic diseases, including obesity, diabetes, and cardiovascular disease.

Despite the transition to agriculture, some populations around the world continued to maintain traditional hunter-gatherer lifestyles, providing valuable insights into the health and dietary habits of our ancestors. Studies of modern hunter-gatherer societies, such as the Hadza of Tanzania and the Inuit of the Arctic, have revealed that these populations exhibit remarkably robust health and low rates of chronic disease, despite consuming diets that differ significantly from modern Western diets.

The dietary patterns of our ancestors offer valuable lessons for contemporary nutrition and health. By understanding the nutritional strategies that allowed our ancestors to thrive in diverse environments, we can glean insights into the types of foods and lifestyle practices that promote optimal health and well-being. Ancestral eating emphasizes consuming whole, nutrient-dense foods that align with our evolutionary heritage, while also incorporating lifestyle factors such as physical activity, adequate sleep, and stress management.

In summary, the evolution of human nutrition is a complex and multifaceted story that reflects the dynamic interplay between our ancestors and their environment. By examining the dietary patterns of our evolutionary predecessors, we can gain valuable insights into the nutritional strategies that shaped human physiology and behavior, and ultimately inform our approach to contemporary nutrition and health.

Examining our evolutionary history

Examining our evolutionary history provides a fascinating insight into the dietary patterns that shaped human physiology and behavior over millions of years. Our journey begins with the emergence of our earliest hominid ancestors, who inhabited East Africa approximately 6 to 7 million years ago. These early hominids, such as Ardipithecus ramidus and Australopithecus afarensis, were primarily herbivorous, subsisting on a diet of fruits, leaves, seeds, and other plant-based foods.

As our ancestors evolved and adapted to new environments, their dietary patterns underwent significant changes. The transition from arboreal to terrestrial life approximately 4 million years ago marked a pivotal moment in human evolution, as our ancestors began to explore new dietary niches and incorporate a wider variety of foods into their diet. With the development of bipedal locomotion and the ability to manipulate objects with their hands, our ancestors became more adept at foraging for food and processing plant materials.

The emergence of Homo habilis approximately 2.5 million years ago marked another important milestone in human evolution, as this species was the first to exhibit stone tool use and tool-making capabilities. These tools enabled our ancestors to access and process a wider range of foods, including meat, marrow, and other animal tissues. The incorporation of animal foods into the diet provided our ancestors with a rich source of protein, fat, and other essential nutrients critical for supporting brain development, reproductive success, and overall health.

Over the course of human evolution, our ancestors continued to adapt to diverse environments and dietary niches, leading to the emergence of a wide range of dietary strategies and adaptations. From the high-fiber, plant-based diets of early hominids to the protein-rich diets of later hominids, our ancestors evolved to thrive on a variety of foods depending on the availability of resources in their environment.

The advent of cooking approximately 2 million years ago further transformed human nutrition, as it allowed our ancestors to access and extract more nutrients from a wider range of foods. Cooking softens plant tissues, making them easier to digest and extract nutrients from, while also reducing the risk of foodborne pathogens and parasites. This technological innovation enabled our ancestors to further diversify their diet and extract more energy from the foods they consumed.

The transition to a more carnivorous diet approximately 2 million years ago marked a significant turning point in human evolution, as it coincided with the emergence of Homo erectus and the expansion of our ancestors' range beyond Africa into Eurasia. The consumption of animal foods provided our ancestors with a reliable and nutrient-dense source of energy, enabling them to thrive in diverse environments and adapt to changing climatic conditions.

The dietary patterns of our ancestors offer valuable insights into the types of foods and nutrients that shaped human physiology and behavior over millions of years of evolution. By understanding our evolutionary history, we can gain a deeper appreciation for the dietary strategies and adaptations that allowed our ancestors to thrive in diverse environments, and ultimately inform our approach to contemporary nutrition and health.

How our ancestors ate and lived

Our ancestors, particularly those from hunter-gatherer societies, lived in close connection with nature, relying on their immediate environment for sustenance and survival. Their dietary patterns and lifestyle were shaped by the resources available to them, as well as their social and cultural practices. Let's delve into how our ancestors ate and lived:

Hunter-Gatherer Lifestyle: Hunter-gatherer societies were nomadic or semi-nomadic, moving with the seasons to follow animal herds, gather seasonal fruits and plants, and access water sources. This lifestyle required constant movement and adaptation to different environments.

Dietary Diversity: Hunter-gatherers consumed a wide variety of foods depending on what was available in their environment. Their diets typically consisted of wild game meats, fish, shellfish, fruits, vegetables, nuts, seeds, roots, and tubers. The diversity of their diet provided a wide array of nutrients essential for optimal health.

Hunting and Gathering: Hunting and gathering were central to the subsistence of hunter-gatherer societies. Men typically hunted large game animals using tools such as spears, bows, and arrows, while women gathered plant foods such as berries, nuts, and roots. Both activities required specialized knowledge of the local environment and the behavior of prey and plant species.

Food Preparation: Our ancestors developed various methods for processing and preparing food to make it more palatable and digestible. This included cooking meat over an open flame to make it safer to eat and easier to digest, as well as pounding and grinding plant foods to extract nutrients and reduce fiber content.

Seasonality: The availability of food varied seasonally, influencing the dietary habits of hunter-gatherer societies. In the spring and summer, when fruits and vegetables were abundant, plant foods made up a larger proportion of their diet. In the fall and winter, when animal migrations occurred and plant foods became scarcer, meat and fish became more prominent in their diet.

Social Structure: Hunter-gatherer societies typically lived in small, egalitarian groups consisting of extended family members. Social structures were often based on cooperation, reciprocity, and sharing, with resources distributed among group members based on need rather than individual ownership.

Connection to Nature: Our ancestors had a deep connection to the natural world, viewing themselves as part of the ecosystem rather than separate from it. They possessed intimate knowledge of their local environment, including the behavior of plants and animals, seasonal patterns, and natural resources.

Cultural Practices: Food acquisition and consumption were often intertwined with cultural practices, rituals, and beliefs. For example, certain foods may have been considered sacred or imbued with spiritual significance, and special ceremonies or feasts may have been held to celebrate successful hunts or harvests.

Overall, the dietary patterns and lifestyle of our ancestors were shaped by their environment, social structure, and cultural practices. Their diet was characterized by diversity, seasonality, and adaptability, providing a blueprint for a balanced and nutritious way of eating that sustained them for millennia. Understanding how our ancestors ate and lived can offer valuable insights into designing a modern diet and lifestyle that promotes optimal health and well-being.

Impact of modern diet

The impact of modern diets on health is profound and far-reaching, contributing to the global burden of chronic diseases such as obesity, diabetes, cardiovascular disease, and certain types of cancer. The shift towards modern dietary patterns, characterized by an overconsumption of processed foods, refined sugars, unhealthy fats, and calorie-dense foods, has led to a range of negative health outcomes. Let's explore the impact of modern diets on health in more detail:

Obesity and Weight Gain: Modern diets high in processed foods, added sugars, and unhealthy fats are major contributors to the global obesity epidemic. These foods are often high in calories and low in essential nutrients, leading to excessive calorie intake and weight gain over time. The rise in obesity rates is associated with an increased risk of numerous health conditions, including type 2 diabetes, heart disease, stroke, and certain types of cancer.

Type 2 Diabetes: The prevalence of type 2 diabetes has risen dramatically in recent decades, largely due to changes in dietary habits and sedentary lifestyles. Modern diets high in refined carbohydrates, added sugars, and processed foods can lead to insulin resistance, a key underlying factor in the development of type 2 diabetes. Poor dietary choices and excessive calorie intake also contribute to obesity, a major risk factor for type 2 diabetes.

Cardiovascular Disease: The consumption of processed foods, trans fats, and excessive amounts of sodium in modern diets is associated with an increased risk of cardiovascular disease, including heart attacks, strokes, and hypertension. These foods contribute to elevated cholesterol levels, high blood pressure, inflammation, and oxidative stress, all of which are risk factors for cardiovascular disease.

Cancer: Certain dietary patterns, such as diets high in processed meats, sugary beverages, and refined carbohydrates, have been linked to an increased risk of certain types of cancer, including colorectal cancer, breast cancer, and pancreatic cancer. Processed meats, in particular, contain harmful additives and carcinogens that can promote the development of cancerous cells in the body.

Nutrient Deficiencies: Modern diets high in processed foods often lack essential nutrients such as vitamins, minerals, fiber, and antioxidants. These foods are often stripped of their natural nutrients during processing and contain added preservatives, additives, and synthetic ingredients. As a result, individuals consuming modern diets may experience nutrient deficiencies, which can impair overall health and increase the risk of chronic diseases.

Gut Health: The composition of modern diets, which are often low in fiber and high in processed foods, can negatively impact gut health. Poor dietary choices can disrupt the balance of beneficial bacteria in the gut microbiome, leading to inflammation, digestive issues, and an increased risk of gastrointestinal disorders such as irritable bowel syndrome (IBS) and inflammatory bowel disease (IBD).

Mental Health: Emerging research suggests that modern diets high in processed foods and unhealthy fats may negatively impact mental health and cognitive function. Diets rich in processed foods, added sugars, and unhealthy fats have been associated with an increased risk of depression, anxiety, and other mood disorders. Conversely, diets rich in whole, nutrient-dense foods such as fruits, vegetables, lean proteins, and healthy fats may support mental well-being and cognitive function.

In summary, modern diets characterized by excessive consumption of processed foods, added sugars, unhealthy fats, and calorie-dense foods have a detrimental impact on health. These dietary patterns contribute to the global burden of chronic diseases, including obesity, diabetes, cardiovascular disease, cancer, and mental health disorders. Understanding the impact of modern diets on health is crucial for promoting healthier dietary choices and addressing the growing prevalence of diet-related diseases in our modern society.

Chapter 3

Principles of the Ancestral Diet

The key principles and guidelines of a healthy diet are essential for promoting optimal health, preventing chronic diseases, and supporting overall well-being. By following these principles, individuals can make informed dietary choices that prioritize nutrient density, balance, and variety. Let's explore some key principles and guidelines for a healthy diet:

Prioritize Whole, Nutrient-Dense Foods: Whole, nutrient-dense foods are the foundation of a healthy diet. These foods are rich in essential nutrients such as vitamins, minerals, antioxidants, and fiber, which are critical for supporting overall health and well-being. Examples include fruits, vegetables, whole grains, lean proteins, nuts, seeds, and legumes.

Focus on Variety and Balance: Consuming a variety of foods from all food groups ensures that you obtain a wide range of nutrients and phytochemicals necessary for optimal health. Aim to include a colorful array of fruits and vegetables, whole grains, lean proteins, and healthy fats in your meals to achieve dietary balance and diversity.

Limit Processed and Ultra-Processed Foods: Processed and ultra-processed foods are often high in added sugars, unhealthy fats, sodium, and artificial additives, while lacking essential nutrients and fiber. These foods contribute to inflammation, oxidative stress, and an increased risk of chronic diseases such as obesity, diabetes, and heart disease. Limit your intake of processed foods, sugary snacks, fast food, and convenience foods, and opt for whole, minimally processed alternatives whenever possible.

Choose Quality Protein Sources: Protein is an essential nutrient that plays a crucial role in building and repairing tissues, supporting immune function, and maintaining muscle mass. Choose lean sources of protein such as poultry, fish, tofu, tempeh, legumes, and nuts, and limit your intake of processed meats and high-fat animal products.

Include Healthy Fats: Healthy fats are an important component of a balanced diet and provide essential fatty acids necessary for brain health, hormone production, and cell membrane function. Include sources of healthy fats such as avocados, nuts, seeds, olive oil, and fatty fish like salmon and mackerel in your meals.

Mindful Eating: Practice mindful eating by paying attention to hunger and fullness cues, eating slowly, and savoring each bite. This can help prevent overeating, promote better digestion, and enhance your overall eating experience.

Stay Hydrated: Hydration is essential for overall health and well-being. Drink plenty of water throughout the day to stay hydrated and support proper bodily functions. Limit your intake of sugary beverages and opt for water, herbal teas, and other hydrating drinks instead.

Moderation is Key: Enjoying foods in moderation is an important aspect of a healthy diet. No single food or nutrient is inherently good or bad, and it's important to strike a balance and practice moderation when it comes to indulgent foods and treats.

Consider Individual Needs and Preferences: Everyone's dietary needs and preferences are unique, and it's important to tailor your diet to meet your individual needs and goals. Consider factors such as age, gender, activity level, food intolerances or allergies, cultural preferences, and personal beliefs when planning your meals.

Plan and Prepare Meals Ahead of Time: Planning and preparing meals ahead of time can help you make healthier food choices, save time and money, and reduce the temptation to rely on convenience foods or takeout. Set aside time each week to plan your meals, create a grocery list, and prepare nutritious meals and snacks to enjoy throughout the week.

By following these key principles and guidelines for a healthy diet, you can make informed dietary choices that promote optimal health, support overall well-being, and enhance your quality of life. Remember to focus on whole, nutrient-dense foods, prioritize variety and balance, and practice moderation and mindful eating to achieve long-term success in maintaining a healthy lifestyle.

Nutrient density and quality of foods

Nutrient density and food quality are fundamental concepts in nutrition that emphasize the importance of choosing foods that provide a high concentration of essential nutrients relative to their calorie content. Nutrient-dense foods are rich in vitamins, minerals, antioxidants, fiber, and other beneficial compounds that are essential for supporting overall health and well-being. Let's explore the concepts of nutrient density and food quality in more detail:

Nutrient Density: Nutrient density refers to the amount of essential nutrients per unit of energy (calories) provided by a food. Foods that are nutrient-dense provide a high concentration of essential nutrients relative to their calorie content, making them valuable sources of nutrition. Examples of nutrient-dense foods include fruits, vegetables, lean proteins, whole grains, nuts, seeds, and legumes. These foods are rich in vitamins, minerals, antioxidants, and fibre, and provide essential nutrients that are necessary for optimal health and well-being.

Benefits of Nutrient-Dense Foods: Consuming a diet rich in nutrient-dense foods offers numerous health benefits. These foods provide essential nutrients that support proper growth and development, immune function, energy metabolism, and overall health. They are also rich in antioxidants and phytochemicals that help protect against chronic diseases such as heart disease, cancer, and diabetes. Additionally, nutrient-dense foods are often high in fiber, which promotes digestive health, regulates blood sugar levels, and helps maintain a healthy weight.

Examples of Nutrient-Dense Foods: Nutrient-dense foods come in a variety of forms and include a wide range of fruits, vegetables, whole grains, lean proteins, nuts, seeds, and legumes. Some examples of nutrient-dense foods include spinach, kale, broccoli, sweet potatoes, berries, oranges, quinoa, brown rice, lean poultry, fish, tofu, almonds, chia seeds, and lentils.

Food Quality: Food quality refers to the overall nutritional value and healthfulness of a food. High-quality foods are minimally processed, free from artificial additives and preservatives, and rich in essential nutrients. They provide a wide range of essential nutrients that are necessary for supporting overall health and well-being. In contrast, low-quality foods are often highly processed, high in added sugars, unhealthy fats, sodium, and artificial additives, while lacking essential nutrients and fiber.

Improving Food Quality: Improving food quality involves making informed dietary choices that prioritize whole, minimally processed foods that are rich in essential nutrients. Choose whole grains over refined grains, fresh fruits and vegetables over canned or processed versions, lean proteins such as poultry, fish, and tofu over processed meats, and healthy fats such as avocados, nuts, and olive oil over trans fats and hydrogenated oils.

Reading Food Labels: Reading food labels can help you determine the nutrient density and quality of foods. Look for foods that are low in added sugars, unhealthy fats, and sodium, and high in essential nutrients such as vitamins, minerals, and fiber. Choose foods with simple, recognizable ingredients and avoid products with long lists of artificial additives and preservatives.

By prioritizing nutrient-dense foods and focusing on food quality, you can make informed dietary choices that support optimal health, prevent chronic diseases, and enhance overall well-being. Incorporating a variety of nutrient-dense foods into your diet and choosing high-quality foods that are minimally processed can help you achieve and maintain a healthy lifestyle.

Understanding macronutrients and micronutrients

Understanding macronutrients and micronutrients is essential for optimizing nutrition and promoting overall health and well-being. These two categories of nutrients play distinct roles in the body and are necessary for supporting various physiological functions. Let's explore the differences between macronutrients and micronutrients, their sources, functions, and recommended intake levels.

Macronutrients:

Macronutrients are nutrients that the body requires in large amounts to provide energy and support basic bodily functions. There are three main categories of macronutrients: carbohydrates, proteins, and fats.

Carbohydrates:
Carbohydrates are the body's primary source of energy and are found in foods such as grains, fruits, vegetables, legumes, and dairy products. They are composed of sugar molecules and come in various forms, including simple sugars (monosaccharides and disaccharides) and complex carbohydrates (polysaccharides).

Functions: Carbohydrates provide energy for the body's cells, particularly the brain and muscles. They are also important for supporting digestive health, regulating blood sugar levels, and providing fiber for bowel regularity.

Sources: Good sources of carbohydrates include whole grains (such as oats, brown rice, quinoa), fruits, vegetables, legumes (such as beans, lentils), and dairy products (such as milk, yogurt).

Proteins:
Proteins are essential for building and repairing tissues, supporting immune function, and regulating various biochemical processes in the body. They are composed of amino acids, which are the building blocks of protein.

Functions: Proteins play a crucial role in the growth and repair of tissues, including muscles, organs, skin, hair, and nails. They also support immune function, enzyme production, hormone regulation, and transportation of molecules within the body.

Sources: Good sources of protein include lean meats (such as chicken, turkey, fish), eggs, dairy products (such as yogurt, cheese), legumes (such as beans, lentils), tofu, tempeh, nuts, and seeds.

Fats:

Fats are essential for providing energy, supporting cell structure and function, and aiding in the absorption of fat-soluble vitamins (such as vitamins A, D, E, and K). They are composed of fatty acids, which can be classified into saturated fats, unsaturated fats (monounsaturated and polyunsaturated fats), and trans fats.

Functions: Fats provide a concentrated source of energy for the body, support the structure and function of cell membranes, and are important for the absorption of fat-soluble vitamins. They also play a role in hormone production, insulation, and protection of organs.

Sources: Good sources of healthy fats include avocados, nuts, seeds, olive oil, fatty fish (such as salmon, mackerel), flaxseeds, chia seeds, and coconut oil.

Micronutrients:

Micronutrients are nutrients that the body requires in smaller amounts but are essential for various physiological functions. They include vitamins and minerals, which play key roles in metabolism, immune function, growth, and development.

Vitamins: Vitamins are organic composites that are essential for colourful metabolic processes in the body. They can be classified into water-answerable vitamins(similar as vitamin C and B vitamins) and fat-answerable vitamins(similar as vitamins A, D, E, and K). Vitamins play a pivotal part in energy metabolism, vulnerable function, antioxidant defence, blood clotting, bone health, and vision. They're involved in multitudinous biochemical responses in the body and are essential for overall health and well- being. Vitamins are set up in a variety of foods, including fruits, vegetables, whole grains, dairy products, spare flesh, fish, nuts, seeds, and fortified foods. It's important to consume a different range of foods to insure an acceptable input of vitamins.

Minerals are inorganic rudiments that are essential for colorful physiological functions in the body. They can be classified into macrominerals(similar as calcium, magnesium, phosphorus, sodium, potassium, and chloride) and trace minerals(similar as iron, zinc, bobby, selenium, iodine, and manganese).

Functions

Minerals play crucial places in bone health, muscle function, whim-wham transmission, fluid balance, enzyme activation, and oxygen transport. They're involved in multitudinous metabolic processes in the body and are essential for maintaining overall health and well-being. Minerals are set up in a variety of foods, including fruits, vegetables, whole grains, dairy products, spare flesh, fish, nuts, seeds, and fortified foods. It's important to consume a different range of foods to ensure an acceptable input of minerals.

Recommended Input situations .

 The recommended input situations for macronutrients and micronutrients vary depending on factors similar as age, gender, exertion position, and specific health conditions. Government health agencies and associations similar as the National Institutes of Health(NIH) and the World Health Organization(WHO) give guidelines and recommendations for nutrient input grounded on scientific substantiation and population health data .

Chapter 4

Benefits of Embracing Ancestral Eating

Improved physical health

Embracing ancestral eating, also known as paleo or primal eating, involves adopting dietary patterns that reflect those of our ancient ancestors. This approach emphasizes consuming whole, minimally processed foods that are thought to align with the dietary habits of our evolutionary predecessors. There are several potential benefits of embracing ancestral eating for improved physical health:

Nutrient Density: Ancestral eating prioritizes nutrient-dense foods such as lean meats, fish, fruits, vegetables, nuts, and seeds. These foods are rich in essential vitamins, minerals, antioxidants, and fiber, providing a wide array of nutrients that support overall health and well-being.

Balanced Macronutrients: Ancestral eating typically involves a balanced intake of macronutrients, including protein, healthy fats, and carbohydrates from whole foods. This balance helps regulate blood sugar levels, promote satiety, and support energy levels throughout the day.

Improved Digestive Health: Ancestral eating emphasizes whole, unprocessed foods that are easier for the body to digest and assimilate. This can promote better digestive health, reduce bloating and discomfort, and support optimal gut microbiome diversity.

Weight Management: Ancestral eating may support weight management and body composition goals by focusing on nutrient-dense foods that promote satiety and reduce cravings for processed and high-calorie foods. Additionally, the emphasis on protein-rich foods can support muscle maintenance and growth, which is important for overall metabolic health.

Reduced Inflammation: Ancestral eating encourages the consumption of anti-inflammatory foods such as fruits, vegetables, nuts, seeds, and omega-3 fatty acids from fatty fish. These foods contain compounds that help reduce systemic inflammation, which is linked to chronic diseases such as heart disease, diabetes, and autoimmune conditions.

Stable Blood Sugar Levels: Ancestral eating emphasizes whole, unprocessed carbohydrates from sources such as fruits, vegetables, and tubers, which have a lower glycemic index compared to refined carbohydrates. This can help stabilize blood sugar levels and reduce the risk of insulin resistance and type 2 diabetes.

Heart Health: Ancestral eating includes foods that are beneficial for heart health, such as fatty fish rich in omega-3 fatty acids, nuts, seeds, and olive oil. These foods help support healthy cholesterol levels, reduce inflammation, and protect against heart disease.

Improved Energy Levels: By focusing on nutrient-dense foods and avoiding processed foods that can cause energy crashes and fatigue, ancestral eating may lead to more stable energy levels throughout the day. This can help improve productivity, mental clarity, and overall well-being.

Supports Natural Circadian Rhythms: Ancestral eating often involves prioritizing whole foods and avoiding artificial additives, preservatives, and excessive caffeine and alcohol consumption. This can support natural circadian rhythms and promote better sleep quality, which is essential for overall health and vitality.

In summary, embracing ancestral eating for improved physical health involves prioritizing nutrient-dense whole foods, balancing macronutrients, supporting digestive health, managing weight, reducing inflammation, stabilizing blood sugar levels, promoting heart health, improving energy levels, and supporting natural circadian rhythms. By adopting dietary patterns that align with our evolutionary heritage, individuals may experience numerous benefits that contribute to overall health and well-being.

Mental clarity and cognitive function

Mental clarity and cognitive function are essential components of overall well-being, encompassing aspects such as memory, focus, concentration, decision-making, and problem-solving abilities. These cognitive functions are influenced by various factors, including genetics, lifestyle habits, environmental factors, and dietary choices. In recent years, there has been growing interest in the impact of nutrition on mental clarity and cognitive function, with emerging research suggesting that certain dietary patterns and nutrients may play a role in supporting brain health and cognitive performance.

Role of Nutrition in Brain Health:
The brain is a highly metabolically active organ that requires a constant supply of nutrients to function optimally. Nutrients such as vitamins, minerals, antioxidants, omega-3 fatty acids, and phytochemicals play crucial roles in supporting brain health and cognitive function. These nutrients are involved in processes such as neurotransmitter synthesis, neuronal communication, neurogenesis, and neuroplasticity, which are essential for maintaining mental clarity and cognitive function throughout life.

Impact of Diet on Cognitive Function:
Research suggests that dietary patterns high in whole, nutrient-dense foods such as fruits, vegetables, whole grains, lean proteins, nuts, seeds, and fatty fish may support cognitive function and reduce the risk of cognitive decline with aging. The Mediterranean diet, for example, which emphasizes plant-based foods, healthy fats, and moderate consumption of fish and poultry, has been associated with better cognitive performance and a lower risk of Alzheimer's disease and dementia.

Inflammation and Cognitive Function:
Chronic inflammation has been implicated in the development of cognitive decline and neurodegenerative diseases such as **Alzheimer's disease.** Certain dietary patterns, such as the Western diet high in processed foods, added sugars, unhealthy fats, and refined carbohydrates, are associated with increased inflammation and oxidative stress, which can negatively impact cognitive function. In contrast, anti-inflammatory diets rich in fruits, vegetables, nuts, seeds, and omega-3 fatty acids have been linked to better cognitive outcomes.

Gut-Brain Axis:
Emerging research suggests that the gut-brain axis, the bidirectional communication pathway between the gut microbiota and the brain, plays a crucial role in regulating cognitive function and mental clarity. The gut microbiota, which consists of trillions of microorganisms residing in the gastrointestinal tract, produce neurotransmitters, metabolites, and other signaling molecules that can influence brain function and behavior. Diet plays a significant role in shaping the composition and diversity of the gut microbiota, highlighting the importance of dietary choices in supporting brain health.

Specific Nutrients and Cognitive Function:
Several nutrients have been studied for their potential role in supporting cognitive function and mental clarity:

Omega-3 fatty acids: Found in fatty fish such as salmon, mackerel, and sardines, as well as walnuts, flaxseeds, and chia seeds, omega-3 fatty acids are essential for brain health and cognitive function. They have been shown to support neuronal membrane integrity, neurotransmitter function, and synaptic plasticity, which are important for memory and learning.

Antioxidants: Found in fruits, vegetables, nuts, seeds, and certain spices, antioxidants such as vitamin C, vitamin E, beta-carotene, and flavonoids help protect the brain from oxidative stress and inflammation, which can contribute to cognitive decline.

B vitamins: Found in whole grains, leafy greens, legumes, nuts, seeds, and animal products, B vitamins such as folate, vitamin B6, and vitamin B12 are involved in neurotransmitter synthesis and methylation processes that are important for cognitive function.

Polyphenols: Found in fruits, vegetables, tea, coffee, cocoa, and red wine, polyphenols have antioxidant and anti-inflammatory properties that may support cognitive function and neuroprotection.

Curcumin: Found in turmeric, curcumin has anti-inflammatory and antioxidant properties that may support cognitive function and protect against neurodegenerative diseases.

Caffeine: Found in coffee, tea, and certain energy drinks, caffeine has been shown to improve alertness, concentration, and cognitive performance in the short term.

Hydration and Cognitive Function:

Proper hydration is essential for supporting cognitive function and mental clarity. Dehydration can impair cognitive performance, attention, and memory, leading to decreased mental clarity and alertness. Drinking an adequate amount of water throughout the day is important for maintaining optimal cognitive function and supporting overall brain health.

Lifestyle Factors:

In addition to nutrition, lifestyle factors such as regular physical activity, adequate sleep, stress management, social engagement, and cognitive stimulation play important roles in maintaining mental clarity and cognitive function. Incorporating these lifestyle habits into daily routines can complement a nutrient-rich diet and support overall brain health.

In conclusion, nutrition plays a crucial role in supporting mental clarity and cognitive function throughout life. By adopting dietary patterns rich in whole, nutrient-dense foods and incorporating specific nutrients known to support brain health, individuals can optimize cognitive performance, reduce the risk of cognitive decline with aging, and promote overall well-being. Additionally, adopting healthy lifestyle habits and managing stress can further support mental clarity and cognitive function in the long term.

Sustainable weight management

Sustainable weight management is a multifaceted approach that focuses on achieving and maintaining a healthy body weight through long-term lifestyle changes that promote overall health and well-being. Unlike short-term fad diets or extreme weight loss strategies, sustainable weight management emphasizes gradual, realistic changes that are maintainable over time. This approach considers not only nutrition and physical activity but also psychological, social, and environmental factors that influence weight and overall health.

Setting Realistic Goals:
Sustainable weight management begins with setting realistic, achievable goals that prioritize overall health and well-being rather than rapid weight loss. Goals should be specific, measurable, achievable, relevant, and time-bound (SMART). Instead of focusing solely on a target weight, consider setting goals related to improving dietary habits, increasing physical activity, managing stress, and improving overall lifestyle habits.

Nutrition and Dietary Habits:
A key component of sustainable weight management is adopting a balanced, nutrient-rich diet that supports overall health and well-being. Instead of restrictive diets or extreme calorie counting, focus on incorporating a variety of nutrient-dense foods such as fruits, vegetables, whole grains, lean proteins, and healthy fats into your meals and snacks. Portion control, mindful eating, and paying attention to hunger and fullness cues can also help promote a healthy relationship with food and support sustainable weight management.

Physical Activity and Exercise:
Regular physical activity is essential for both weight management and overall health. Aim for a combination of aerobic exercise, strength training, and flexibility exercises to improve cardiovascular health, build lean muscle mass, and increase metabolism. Find activities that you enjoy and can incorporate into your daily routine, whether it's walking, cycling, swimming, dancing, or participating in group fitness classes. Aim for at least 150 minutes of moderate-intensity aerobic activity or 75 minutes of vigorous-intensity aerobic activity per week, along with muscle-strengthening activities on two or more days per week.

Behavioral Strategies:
Sustainable weight management involves adopting behavioral strategies that support healthy eating habits and lifestyle changes. This includes strategies such as meal planning and preparation, mindful eating, keeping a food journal, practicing portion control, and setting SMART goals. Identifying triggers for unhealthy eating habits, such as stress, boredom, or emotional eating, and finding alternative coping mechanisms can also support long-term success.

Mindfulness and Stress Management:
Stress management and mindfulness techniques can play a crucial role in sustainable weight management by reducing emotional eating and promoting self-awareness. Incorporate stress-reducing activities into your daily routine, such as mindfulness meditation, deep breathing exercises, yoga, tai chi, or spending time in nature. Prioritizing adequate sleep, practicing relaxation techniques, and seeking social support can also help manage stress and support overall well-being.

Social Support and Accountability:
Having a support system in place can significantly impact your success in sustainable weight management. Seek support from friends, family members, or a support group who can provide encouragement, accountability, and motivation along your journey. Consider joining a weight management program, online community, or working with a registered dietitian or health coach who can provide guidance, support, and accountability.

Environmental Factors:
Environmental factors such as access to healthy food options, built environment, social norms, and cultural influences can influence dietary habits and physical activity levels. Making changes to your environment that support healthy choices, such as keeping healthy snacks readily available, creating a supportive home environment, and finding opportunities for physical activity in your community, can help facilitate sustainable weight management.

Lifelong Approach:
Sustainable weight management is not a quick fix or temporary solution but rather a lifelong commitment to health and well-being. Focus on making gradual, sustainable changes to your habits and behaviors that you can maintain over time. Celebrate small victories along the way and be patient with yourself as you progress toward your goals. Remember that sustainable weight management is about progress, not perfection, and focus on building healthy habits that last a lifetime.

In conclusion, sustainable weight management is a holistic approach that encompasses nutrition, physical activity, behavioral strategies, stress management, social support, and environmental factors. By adopting realistic goals, making gradual lifestyle changes, and prioritizing overall health and well-being, individuals can achieve and maintain a healthy body weight in a sustainable manner. Remember that sustainable weight management is not a one-size-fits-all approach, and it's important to find strategies and techniques that work best for you and support your long-term health goals.

Chapter 5

Common Misconceptions and Debates

Addressing myths and misconceptions

Addressing myths and misconceptions about health and wellness is essential for promoting accurate information, encouraging evidence-based practices, and supporting informed decision-making among individuals. Myths and misconceptions often arise from a variety of sources, including cultural beliefs, anecdotal evidence, misinformation spread through media channels, and the promotion of fad diets or pseudoscientific claims. These myths can perpetuate harmful practices, undermine public health efforts, and contribute to confusion surrounding health-related topics. Let's explore some common myths and misconceptions and provide evidence-based explanations to debunk them:

Myth: Carbohydrates are inherently bad for you
This myth stems from the misconception that all carbohydrates are equal and contribute to weight gain and health issues. While it's true that excessive consumption of refined carbohydrates and added sugars can lead to health problems such as obesity and insulin resistance, not all carbohydrates are bad for you. Carbohydrates are an essential macronutrient that provides the body with energy, and they can be found in a variety of nutrient-dense foods such as fruits, vegetables, whole grains, and legumes. These whole food sources of carbohydrates are rich in fiber, vitamins, minerals, and phytochemicals, and they play a crucial role in supporting overall health and well-being.

Myth: Fat-free and low-fat foods are always healthier
This myth stems from the belief that reducing fat intake is necessary for weight loss and improving heart health. While it's important to limit intake of unhealthy fats such as trans fats and excessive saturated fats, not all fats are unhealthy. In fact, certain types of healthy fats, such as monounsaturated and polyunsaturated fats found in foods like avocados, nuts, seeds, and fatty fish, are beneficial for heart health and overall well-being. Additionally, many fat-free and low-fat foods contain added sugars, artificial additives, and refined carbohydrates to compensate for the lack of fat, which can be detrimental to health. It's important to focus on the overall nutritional quality of foods rather than solely relying on fat content.

Myth: Eating late at night causes weight gain
This myth suggests that consuming food late at night leads to weight gain because the body's metabolism slows down during sleep. While it's true that consuming excessive calories late at night can contribute to weight gain, the timing of meals and snacks is less important than the total amount and quality of calories consumed throughout the day. What matters most is maintaining a balanced diet and managing portion sizes, regardless of the time of day. It's important to listen to your body's hunger and fullness cues and make mindful choices about when and what to eat.

Myth: You can spot-reduce fat from specific areas of the body
This myth suggests that performing targeted exercises or using specific products can reduce fat from specific areas of the body, such as the abdomen, thighs, or arms. However, spot reduction is a myth, and it's not possible to selectively lose fat from specific areas of the body through exercise or targeted treatments. Fat loss occurs throughout the body in response to overall calorie deficit and energy expenditure. To reduce body fat and improve body composition, it's important to focus on overall weight loss through a combination of regular physical activity, balanced nutrition, and lifestyle modifications.

Myth: Detox diets and cleanses are necessary for removing toxins from the body
This myth suggests that detox diets and cleanses are necessary for removing toxins from the body and promoting health and weight loss. However, there is little scientific evidence to support the effectiveness of detox diets and cleanses for removing toxins or improving health outcomes. The body has its own natural detoxification processes, primarily carried out by the liver, kidneys, and lymphatic system, which are capable of removing waste products and toxins from the body. Instead of relying on extreme detox programs, focus on adopting a balanced diet rich in whole, nutrient-dense foods, staying hydrated, getting regular exercise, and prioritizing adequate sleep to support the body's natural detoxification processes.

Myth: All-natural and organic foods are always healthier
This myth suggests that all-natural and organic foods are inherently healthier and superior to conventionally grown or processed foods. While organic foods may have certain benefits, such as being free from synthetic pesticides and additives, not all natural or organic foods are healthier than their conventional counterparts. It's important to focus on the overall nutritional quality of foods rather than solely relying on labels like "natural" or "organic." Additionally, organic foods may be more expensive and not always accessible to everyone, so it's important to prioritize budget-friendly and accessible options that align with your dietary preferences and values.

Myth: Supplements can replace a balanced diet
This myth suggests that dietary supplements are necessary for meeting nutritional needs and can replace the need for a balanced diet. While dietary supplements can be useful for filling nutrient gaps in certain populations, they should not be seen as a substitute for a balanced diet. Whole foods provide a wide range of essential nutrients, fiber, and phytochemicals that work synergistically to support overall health and well-being. Supplements are not regulated

in the same way as food and drugs, and taking high doses of certain vitamins and minerals can be harmful. It's best to focus on obtaining nutrients from whole foods whenever possible and consult with a healthcare professional before taking supplements.

In conclusion, addressing myths and misconceptions about health and wellness is essential for promoting accurate information, encouraging evidence-based practices, and supporting informed decision-making among individuals. By debunking common myths and providing evidence-based explanations, we can empower individuals to make informed choices about their health and well-being and promote positive behavior change that supports long-term health outcomes. It's important to critically evaluate sources of information, seek out evidence-based resources, and consult with healthcare professionals or registered dietitians for personalized guidance and support.

Debates within the ancestral eating community

The ancestral eating community encompasses individuals who advocate for dietary patterns that reflect those of our ancient ancestors, often referred to as the paleo or primal diet. While there is general consensus within the ancestral eating community about the importance of consuming whole, minimally processed foods and prioritizing nutrient-dense options, there are also debates and disagreements regarding specific aspects of ancestral eating. These debates revolve around various topics, including macronutrient ratios, food choices, agricultural practices, ethical considerations, and the interpretation of evolutionary biology and anthropology. Let's explore some of the key debates within the ancestral eating community:

Macronutrient Ratios:
One of the ongoing debates within the ancestral eating community revolves around the ideal macronutrient ratios for optimal health. While ancestral eating advocates generally agree on the importance of prioritizing whole foods and avoiding processed carbohydrates and refined sugars, there is disagreement about the optimal ratio of carbohydrates, proteins, and fats in the diet. Some proponents advocate for a higher-fat, moderate-protein, low-carbohydrate approach, citing evolutionary and anthropological evidence suggesting that our ancestors consumed diets higher in fat and protein and lower in carbohydrates. Others argue for a more balanced approach that includes a moderate intake of all three macronutrients, emphasizing the importance of individual variability and metabolic flexibility.

Food Choices:
Another debate within the ancestral eating community centers around specific food choices and whether certain foods should be included or excluded from an ancestral diet. While there is general agreement about the importance of consuming nutrient-dense whole foods such as fruits, vegetables, meats, seafood, nuts, and seeds, there is disagreement about the inclusion of certain foods that were not available to our ancestors, such as dairy products, grains, and legumes. Some proponents argue that these foods can be included in moderation as part of a balanced ancestral diet, while others advocate for strict avoidance based on concerns about potential negative health effects, such as inflammation, gut irritation, and autoimmune reactions.

Agricultural Practices:
The ancestral eating community also debates the impact of modern agricultural practices on the nutritional quality of food and its compatibility with an ancestral diet. Some proponents argue for the consumption of foods that are organically grown, locally sourced, and produced using sustainable farming methods, citing concerns about the use of synthetic pesticides, genetically modified organisms (GMOs), and industrial farming practices. Others argue that the focus should be on the nutritional quality of food rather than specific agricultural practices, emphasizing the importance of consuming nutrient-dense whole foods regardless of how they are produced.

Ethical Considerations:
Ethical considerations also play a role in debates within the ancestral eating community, particularly regarding the sourcing and consumption of animal products. While many proponents of ancestral eating advocate for the inclusion of animal products such as meat, poultry, fish, and eggs in the diet due to their nutrient density and role in human evolution, others raise concerns about the ethical implications of animal agriculture, including animal welfare, environmental sustainability, and the ethical treatment of animals. Some proponents advocate for ethical sourcing practices such as pasture-raised, grass-fed, and organic animal products, while others argue for plant-based or vegan variations of the ancestral diet that exclude animal products altogether.

Interpretation of Evolutionary Biology and Anthropology:
Debates within the ancestral eating community also extend to the interpretation of evolutionary biology and anthropology and how these disciplines inform dietary recommendations. While proponents of ancestral eating generally agree that our evolutionary history provides valuable insights into our dietary needs and preferences, there is disagreement about the extent to which modern humans should emulate the dietary habits of our ancient ancestors. Some proponents advocate for strict adherence to a paleolithic diet based on evolutionary principles, while others argue for a more flexible approach that incorporates modern scientific research and acknowledges the evolutionary adaptations that have occurred in human populations over time.

Nutrient Density vs. Macronutrient Ratios:
Another debate within the ancestral eating community revolves around the relative
importance of nutrient density versus macronutrient ratios in promoting optimal health. While
both nutrient density and macronutrient ratios are important factors to consider in dietary
recommendations, there is disagreement about which should take precedence. Some
proponents argue that prioritizing nutrient-dense whole foods is the most important aspect of
an ancestral diet, regardless of specific macronutrient ratios. Others argue that macronutrient
ratios play a crucial role in metabolic health and weight management and should be carefully
balanced to optimize health outcomes.

Individual Variability and Personalization:
Finally, debates within the ancestral eating community also center around the concept of
individual variability and the importance of personalized dietary recommendations. While
there are general guidelines and principles that apply to ancestral eating, there is recognition
that individual dietary needs and preferences can vary based on factors such as genetics,
metabolism, activity level, and health status. Some proponents advocate for a one-size-fits-all
approach to ancestral eating, while others argue for a more personalized approach that takes
into account individual differences and allows for flexibility in dietary choices.

In conclusion, the ancestral eating community is characterized by a diversity of opinions and
perspectives, leading to ongoing debates and discussions about various aspects of ancestral
eating. While there is general agreement about the importance of prioritizing whole,
minimally processed foods and incorporating evolutionary principles into dietary
recommendations, there is also disagreement about specific macronutrient ratios, food
choices, agricultural practices, ethical considerations, interpretation of evolutionary biology
and anthropology, and the relative importance of nutrient density versus macronutrient ratios.
These debates highlight the complexity of dietary recommendations and the ongoing
evolution of our understanding of nutrition and human health.

Science versus anecdotal evidence

The debate between science and anecdotal evidence is a longstanding and complex issue that
arises in various fields, including medicine, nutrition, psychology, and social sciences. In the
context of health and wellness, this debate centers around the relative value and validity of
scientific research versus individual experiences and anecdotal reports in shaping our
understanding of health-related topics. While both science and anecdotal evidence can
provide valuable insights, they differ in their methodologies, reliability, and generalizability.
Let's explore the characteristics of science and anecdotal evidence, their respective strengths
and limitations, and how they intersect in shaping our understanding of health and wellness.

Science:

Science refers to the systematic study of the natural world through observation, experimentation, and the formulation of testable hypotheses. It relies on rigorous methodologies, peer review, and empirical evidence to establish reliable knowledge and understanding of phenomena. In the context of health and wellness, scientific research encompasses various disciplines, including biology, physiology, biochemistry, epidemiology, and psychology. Here are some key characteristics of scientific research:

Empirical Evidence: Scientific research relies on empirical evidence obtained through observation, experimentation, and data collection. This evidence is subject to systematic analysis and interpretation, allowing researchers to draw conclusions and make evidence-based recommendations.

Rigorous Methodologies: Scientific studies employ rigorous methodologies to ensure validity, reliability, and reproducibility of results. This includes randomized controlled trials, longitudinal studies, cohort studies, case-control studies, and meta-analyses, among others.

Peer Review: Scientific research undergoes peer review, where experts in the field critically evaluate the study design, methodology, results, and conclusions before publication in peer-reviewed journals. Peer review helps ensure the quality and integrity of research findings.

Generalizability: Scientific research aims to produce generalizable findings that can be applied to broader populations or contexts. This requires careful sampling, statistical analysis, and consideration of confounding variables to ensure the validity and generalizability of results.

Cumulative Knowledge: Scientific research contributes to a cumulative body of knowledge, where new findings build upon existing evidence and theories. This iterative process allows for the refinement and advancement of scientific understanding over time.

Anecdotal Evidence:

Anecdotal evidence refers to individual accounts, personal experiences, testimonials, and stories that provide subjective perspectives on a particular phenomenon or topic. Unlike scientific research, anecdotal evidence is not based on systematic observation, experimentation, or empirical data collection. Instead, it relies on personal observations, perceptions, and interpretations of individuals' experiences. Here are some key characteristics of anecdotal evidence:

Subjective Nature: Anecdotal evidence is inherently subjective, reflecting the personal perspectives, beliefs, and experiences of individuals. It is influenced by factors such as memory bias, selective perception, and individual differences in perception and interpretation.

Limited Scope: Anecdotal evidence is typically based on individual or small-scale experiences, making it limited in scope and generalizability. It does not provide a comprehensive or representative view of a phenomenon and may be influenced by unique circumstances or outliers.

Confirmation Bias: Anecdotal evidence is susceptible to confirmation bias, where individuals selectively recall or emphasize experiences that confirm their pre-existing beliefs or hypotheses. This can lead to an overestimation of the validity or significance of anecdotal reports.

Lack of Control: Anecdotal evidence lacks the control and standardization of scientific research, making it difficult to isolate specific variables or establish causality. Without systematic experimentation or rigorous methodologies, anecdotal reports may be influenced by confounding factors or alternative explanations.

Role of Placebo Effect: Anecdotal evidence may be influenced by the placebo effect, where individuals experience perceived improvements in health or well-being due to psychological or placebo responses rather than the intervention itself. This can contribute to the perceived effectiveness of certain interventions or treatments based on anecdotal reports.

Intersection of Science and Anecdotal Evidence:

While science and anecdotal evidence represent distinct approaches to understanding health and wellness, they are not mutually exclusive. In fact, they often intersect and complement each other in shaping our understanding of complex health-related topics. Here are some ways in which science and anecdotal evidence intersect:

Hypothesis Generation: Anecdotal evidence can serve as a starting point for hypothesis generation in scientific research. Observations and reports of unusual or unexpected outcomes may prompt researchers to investigate further through systematic experimentation and empirical observation.

Clinical Observation: Anecdotal evidence plays a role in clinical practice and patient care, where healthcare providers rely on patient-reported symptoms, experiences, and responses to treatment to inform diagnosis and treatment decisions. While individual anecdotes may not constitute scientific evidence, they can provide valuable insights into patient experiences and preferences.

Pilot Studies: Anecdotal evidence can inform the design and implementation of pilot studies or feasibility studies, which serve as preliminary investigations to assess the viability and potential efficacy of interventions before conducting large-scale scientific research.

Qualitative Research: Anecdotal evidence is often used in qualitative research methods, such as interviews, focus groups, and case studies, to explore subjective experiences, perceptions, and narratives related to health and wellness. Qualitative research complements quantitative research by providing rich, detailed insights into individuals' lived experiences and perspectives.

Patient-Centered Care: Anecdotal evidence can inform patient-centered care approaches that prioritize individual preferences, values, and experiences in healthcare decision-making. Healthcare providers may incorporate patient-reported outcomes and anecdotal reports into shared decision-making processes to tailor treatment plans to individual needs and preferences.

Conclusion:

The debate between science and anecdotal evidence underscores the complexity of understanding health and wellness. While scientific research provides a rigorous and systematic approach to generating evidence-based knowledge, anecdotal evidence offers subjective perspectives and personal experiences that can complement and enrich our understanding of complex health-related topics. Both approaches have their strengths and limitations, and they often intersect and inform each other in shaping our understanding of health and wellness. By recognizing the value of both science and anecdotal evidence, we can foster a more comprehensive and nuanced approach to promoting health and well-being

Chapter 6

Implementing the Ancestral Diet: Practical Tips and Guidance

Transitioning to an ancestral diet involves adopting a dietary approach that reflects the eating habits of our ancient ancestors, focusing on whole, minimally processed foods that are nutrient-dense and support optimal health. This dietary shift is often referred to as the paleo or primal diet and is based on the premise that our bodies are genetically adapted to thrive on the foods that our ancestors consumed during the Paleolithic era.

Understanding Ancestral Eating:
Ancestral eating is based on the idea that our bodies are best suited to the foods that our ancestors consumed before the advent of agriculture and modern processed foods. During the Paleolithic era, our ancestors primarily relied on hunting and gathering to obtain their food, consuming a diet that was rich in lean meats, fish, fruits, vegetables, nuts, and seeds. This diet provided a balanced intake of macronutrients (protein, fat, and carbohydrates) and a wide array of essential vitamins, minerals, and antioxidants.

Principles of Ancestral Eating:
The principles of ancestral eating revolve around consuming whole, nutrient-dense foods while avoiding processed and refined foods that were not available to our ancestors. Key principles of ancestral eating include:

Prioritizing whole foods: Focus on consuming foods that are minimally processed and as close to their natural state as possible. This includes fresh fruits and vegetables, lean meats, fish, poultry, nuts, seeds, and healthy fats.

Eliminating processed foods: Avoid foods that are highly processed, including refined grains, added sugars, artificial additives, and hydrogenated oils. These foods are often low in nutrients and can contribute to inflammation and chronic diseases.

Emphasizing nutrient density: Choose foods that are rich in essential nutrients such as vitamins, minerals, antioxidants, and phytochemicals. These nutrients support overall health, immune function, and vitality.

Balancing macronutrients: Aim for a balanced intake of protein, fat, and carbohydrates from whole food sources. This helps regulate blood sugar levels, support satiety, and provide sustained energy throughout the day.

Incorporating variety: Include a variety of foods in your diet to ensure a diverse range of nutrients and flavors. Experiment with different fruits, vegetables, meats, and spices to keep meals interesting and satisfying.

Transitioning to an Ancestral Diet:
Transitioning to an ancestral diet is a gradual process that involves making small, sustainable changes to your eating habits over time. Here are some steps to help you transition to an ancestral diet:

Educate yourself: Learn about the principles of ancestral eating and the types of foods that are included in this dietary approach. Familiarize yourself with the foods that our ancestors would have consumed and why they are considered beneficial for health.

Assess your current diet: Take stock of your current eating habits and identify areas where you can make improvements. Pay attention to the types of foods you typically consume and consider how they align with the principles of ancestral eating.

Make gradual changes: Start by making small, manageable changes to your diet. For example, replace processed snacks with whole food options like fruits, vegetables, nuts, and seeds. Gradually reduce your intake of processed foods and replace them with nutrient-dense alternatives.

Focus on whole foods: Shift your focus towards incorporating more whole, minimally processed foods into your meals. Include a variety of fruits, vegetables, lean meats, fish, poultry, nuts, seeds, and healthy fats in your diet.

Experiment with new recipes: Explore new recipes and cooking techniques that align with the principles of ancestral eating. Look for paleo or primal recipes that feature whole food ingredients and experiment with different flavors and cuisines.

Listen to your body: Pay attention to how different foods make you feel and adjust your diet accordingly. Notice how your energy levels, digestion, and overall well-being are affected by the foods you eat.

Seek support: Connect with others who are following an ancestral diet for support and inspiration. Join online communities, forums, or social media groups where you can share experiences, ask questions, and find encouragement along your journey.

Challenges and Tips:
Transitioning to an ancestral diet may pose some challenges, especially if you are accustomed to a diet that is high in processed foods. Here are some common challenges and tips for overcoming them:

Cravings for processed foods: You may experience cravings for processed foods, especially if they were a regular part of your diet. Combat cravings by focusing on nutrient-dense whole foods that satisfy your hunger and provide sustained energy.
Social situations: Social situations, such as dining out or attending social gatherings, may present challenges when following an ancestral diet. Plan ahead by researching restaurant menus, bringing your own dishes to potlucks, or politely explaining your dietary preferences to hosts.

Convenience and accessibility: Convenience foods that are high in processed ingredients may be more readily available than whole, minimally processed options. Plan ahead by preparing meals and snacks in advance, stocking your pantry with staple ingredients, and seeking out local markets or farm stands for fresh produce.

Personal preferences and taste preferences: Not everyone enjoys the same foods, and personal taste preferences may influence your ability to adhere to an ancestral diet. Experiment with different foods, flavors, and cooking techniques to find options that you enjoy and look forward to eating.
Benefits of an Ancestral Diet:
Transitioning to an ancestral diet can offer numerous benefits for your health and well-being, including:

Improved nutrient intake: An ancestral diet prioritizes nutrient-dense whole foods that provide essential vitamins, minerals, antioxidants, and phytochemicals that support overall health and vitality.
Better digestion: Whole foods are often easier for the body to digest and assimilate compared to processed foods, leading to improved digestion and gut health.

Stable energy levels: An ancestral diet focuses on balanced macronutrient intake from whole food sources, which can help regulate blood sugar levels and provide sustained energy throughout the day.

Weight management: An ancestral diet emphasizes nutrient-dense whole foods and balanced macronutrient intake, which can support healthy weight management and body composition.

Reduced inflammation: An ancestral diet eliminates processed foods that are high in inflammatory ingredients such as refined sugars, artificial additives, and hydrogenated oils, which can help reduce inflammation in the body.

Enhanced well-being: Many individuals report improvements in overall well-being, including increased energy, better mood, and improved sleep, when following an ancestral diet.

In conclusion, transitioning to an ancestral diet involves adopting a dietary approach that prioritizes whole, minimally processed foods that are nutrient-dense and support optimal health. This dietary shift is based on the premise that our bodies are genetically adapted to thrive on the foods that our ancestors consumed during the Paleolithic era. By gradually making changes to your eating habits, focusing on whole foods, experimenting with new recipes, and seeking support from others, you can successfully transition to an ancestral diet and experience the numerous benefits it has to offer for your health and well-being.

Meal planning and preparation

Meal planning and preparation are essential components of a healthy lifestyle, providing numerous benefits such as saving time and money, reducing food waste, supporting dietary goals, and promoting overall well-being. Whether you're following a specific dietary approach like the ancestral diet or simply aiming to eat healthier, meal planning and preparation can help you make nutritious and delicious meals while minimizing stress and decision fatigue. In this comprehensive guide, we'll explore the importance of meal planning and preparation, practical tips for getting started, and strategies for success.

Why Meal Planning and Preparation Matter:

Time-Saving: Meal planning and preparation can save you time throughout the week by reducing the need to make last-minute trips to the grocery store or decide what to eat for each meal. By planning ahead, you can streamline your grocery shopping, cooking, and mealtime routines, freeing up time for other activities.

Cost-Effective: Planning your meals in advance allows you to make strategic decisions about your grocery purchases, helping you stick to your budget and avoid impulse buys. Additionally, cooking at home is generally more affordable than dining out, so meal planning and preparation can help you save money in the long run.

Reduced Food Waste: When you plan your meals in advance, you're less likely to overbuy or let ingredients go to waste. By creating a shopping list based on your meal plan and using up ingredients before they spoil, you can minimize food waste and save money on groceries.

Healthier Choices: Meal planning and preparation empower you to make healthier food choices by allowing you to incorporate a variety of nutrient-dense ingredients into your meals. When you plan your meals ahead of time, you can ensure that you're meeting your nutritional needs and avoiding the temptation of unhealthy convenience foods.

Portion Control: Planning your meals in advance can help you practice portion control and prevent overeating. By portioning out your meals and snacks ahead of time, you can avoid mindless eating and stay on track with your dietary goals.

Stress Reduction: Meal planning and preparation can help reduce stress and decision fatigue associated with mealtime. When you have a plan in place, you can approach mealtime with confidence, knowing that you have nutritious and satisfying options available.

Getting Started with Meal Planning:

Set Goals and Priorities: Before you begin meal planning, take some time to reflect on your dietary goals, preferences, and lifestyle. Consider factors such as your nutritional needs, dietary restrictions, budget, and schedule when planning your meals.

Choose a Method: There are various methods for meal planning, so choose one that works best for you. Some options include planning your meals for the week ahead, batch cooking and freezing meals for later, or using a meal delivery service.

Create a Meal Calendar: Start by creating a meal calendar for the week, outlining what you'll eat for breakfast, lunch, dinner, and snacks each day. Consider factors such as convenience, variety, and balance when planning your meals.

Inventory Your Pantry and Fridge: Before you create your meal plan and grocery list, take inventory of what you already have on hand in your pantry and fridge. This will help you avoid duplicate purchases and ensure that you use up ingredients before they expire.

Plan Your Meals: Once you've assessed your needs and inventory, start planning your meals for the week. Consider incorporating a variety of protein sources, vegetables, fruits, whole grains, and healthy fats into your meals to ensure a balanced diet.

Create a Grocery List: Based on your meal plan, create a grocery list of the ingredients you'll need for the week. Organize your list by category (e.g., produce, dairy, proteins) to make shopping more efficient.

Shop with Purpose: Armed with your meal plan and grocery list, head to the store to stock up on ingredients for the week. Stick to your list as much as possible to avoid impulse buys and stay within your budget.

Tips for Successful Meal Preparation:

Set Aside Time: Schedule dedicated time each week for meal preparation. Whether it's a few hours on Sunday afternoon or an evening during the week, setting aside time for meal prep will help you stay organized and on track.

Batch Cook: Consider batch cooking staple ingredients such as grains, proteins, and vegetables in large quantities to use throughout the week. Batch cooking saves time and allows you to mix and match ingredients to create a variety of meals.

Prep Ingredients: Wash, chop, and portion out ingredients in advance to streamline meal preparation. Having prepped ingredients on hand makes it easier to throw together meals quickly during the week.

Use Time-Saving Appliances: Invest in time-saving kitchen appliances such as a slow cooker, Instant Pot, or air fryer to simplify meal preparation. These appliances can help you cook meals more efficiently and with less hands-on time.

Store Meals Properly: Once your meals are prepared, portion them out into individual containers and store them in the fridge or freezer. Proper storage ensures that your meals stay fresh and safe to eat throughout the week.

Label and Date: To keep track of your meals and prevent food waste, label your containers with the contents and date of preparation. This will help you identify meals quickly and ensure that you use them before they spoil.

Rotate Your Menu: To prevent boredom and ensure variety in your meals, rotate your menu regularly and experiment with new recipes and flavors. Incorporate seasonal produce and culinary inspiration to keep your meals interesting.

Overcoming Common Challenges:

Time Constraints: If you're short on time, prioritize quick and easy meal options such as one-pot meals, sheet pan dinners, or make-ahead salads. Look for shortcuts such as pre-cut vegetables or pre-cooked proteins to streamline meal preparation.

Lack of Inspiration: If you're struggling with meal ideas, seek inspiration from cookbooks, food blogs, or meal planning apps. Consider joining online communities or social media groups where you can share recipes and meal ideas with others.

Limited Kitchen Skills: If you're new to meal planning and preparation, start with simple recipes and gradually build your cooking skills over time. Look for beginner-friendly recipes with minimal ingredients and step-by-step instructions.

Budget Constraints: If you're on a tight budget, focus on budget-friendly ingredients such as beans, lentils, whole grains, and seasonal produce. Look for sales, discounts, and coupons to save money on groceries, and consider buying in bulk to save on staple items.

Family Preferences: If you're cooking for a family with different preferences and dietary needs, consider involving them in the meal planning process. Offer a variety of options and allow everyone to customize their meals to suit their tastes.

Sustainability: If you're concerned about sustainability, prioritize locally sourced, seasonal ingredients and reduce food waste by using up leftovers and incorporating scraps into your meals. Consider meal planning and preparation as a way to reduce your environmental impact and support sustainable food practices.

Conclusion:

Meal planning and preparation are valuable tools for achieving your dietary goals, saving time and money, and promoting overall well-being. By taking the time to plan your meals in advance, create a grocery list, and prepare meals ahead of time, you can streamline your cooking routine, make healthier choices, and enjoy delicious and satisfying meals throughout the week. With the right strategies and a bit of planning, meal planning and preparation can become an enjoyable and sustainable part of your healthy lifestyle.

Overcoming challenges and setbacks

Overcoming challenges and setbacks is an inevitable part of any journey, including when it comes to adopting a healthier lifestyle through meal planning and preparation. While challenges and setbacks may arise, they can also serve as opportunities for growth, learning, and resilience. In this section, we'll explore common challenges and setbacks that individuals may encounter during meal planning and preparation, as well as strategies for overcoming them.

Common Challenges and Setbacks:

Time Constraints: One of the most common challenges individuals face when it comes to meal planning and preparation is finding the time to do so. Busy schedules, work commitments, and family responsibilities can make it difficult to dedicate time to meal planning and preparation.

Lack of Motivation: Another challenge is a lack of motivation or consistency in sticking to a meal planning and preparation routine. It's common to feel overwhelmed or unmotivated, especially when faced with competing priorities or fatigue.

Limited Cooking Skills: Some individuals may struggle with limited cooking skills or confidence in the kitchen, which can hinder their ability to plan and prepare meals effectively.

Budget Constraints: Budget constraints can also pose a challenge, as individuals may feel restricted in their ability to purchase healthy ingredients or invest in kitchen tools and equipment.

Family Preferences: Balancing the preferences and dietary needs of family members can be challenging, especially if there are varying tastes, preferences, or dietary restrictions to accommodate.

Environmental Factors: External factors such as access to grocery stores, availability of fresh produce, and kitchen facilities can also impact meal planning and preparation efforts.

Strategies for Overcoming Challenges and Setbacks:

Set Realistic Goals: Start by setting realistic and achievable goals for your meal planning and preparation efforts. Break down larger goals into smaller, manageable tasks, and celebrate your progress along the way.

Prioritize Self-Care: Prioritize self-care and carve out dedicated time for meal planning and preparation in your schedule. Treat meal preparation as an act of self-care and nourishment, rather than a chore or obligation.

Simplify Where Possible: Simplify your meal planning and preparation process by focusing on quick and easy recipes, batch cooking, and using time-saving kitchen tools and appliances.

Build Cooking Skills: Invest time in building your cooking skills and confidence in the kitchen. Start with basic cooking techniques and gradually experiment with new recipes and flavors to expand your culinary repertoire.

Involve Family Members: Involve family members in the meal planning and preparation process to foster a sense of ownership and collaboration. Consider holding family meetings to discuss meal preferences, plan menus together, and assign tasks.

Embrace Flexibility: Embrace flexibility in your meal planning and preparation efforts. Recognize that not every meal will go according to plan, and that's okay. Be willing to adapt and adjust as needed, and don't be too hard on yourself if things don't go perfectly.

Seek Support: Reach out for support from friends, family, or online communities who share similar goals or experiences. Share your challenges and setbacks openly, and seek advice, encouragement, and accountability from others.

Celebrate Small Wins: Celebrate your successes, no matter how small. Acknowledge your efforts and progress, and celebrate the positive changes you've made towards a healthier lifestyle.

Practice Self-Compassion: Be kind to yourself and practice self-compassion during times of challenge or setback. Remember that setbacks are a natural part of the process, and they provide opportunities for learning and growth.

Reflect and Learn: Take time to reflect on your challenges and setbacks, and identify any patterns or lessons learned. Use setbacks as opportunities for reflection and learning, and adjust your approach as needed moving forward.

In conclusion, overcoming challenges and setbacks is an essential part of the meal planning and preparation journey. By setting realistic goals, prioritizing self-care, building cooking skills, involving family members, embracing flexibility, seeking support, celebrating small wins, practicing self-compassion, and reflecting and learning from setbacks, you can navigate challenges effectively and continue on your path towards a healthier lifestyle. Remember that progress is not always linear, and setbacks are opportunities for growth and resilience. Keep moving forward, and don't be afraid to ask for help when needed.

Chapter 7

Recipes Inspired by Our Ancestors

Recipes inspired by our ancestors draw inspiration from the dietary habits of our ancient predecessors, focusing on whole, minimally processed ingredients that nourish the body and support optimal health. These recipes prioritize nutrient-dense foods such as lean meats, fish, poultry, fruits, vegetables, nuts, seeds, and healthy fats, while avoiding processed grains, sugars, and artificial additives. By incorporating ingredients that were available to our ancestors during the Paleolithic era, these recipes offer a delicious and satisfying way to embrace ancestral eating principles. Let's explore breakfast, lunch, dinner, and snack recipes inspired by our ancestors:

Breakfast, lunch, dinner, and snack recipes

Breakfast Recipes:

Paleo Omelette: Start your day with a hearty and protein-packed omelette made with pasture-raised eggs and a variety of fresh vegetables. Sauté diced onions, bell peppers, mushrooms, and spinach in olive oil until tender. Whisk together eggs and pour over the vegetables, cooking until set. Fold the omelette in half and serve with sliced avocado and a sprinkle of fresh herbs.

Sweet Potato Hash: Enjoy a satisfying and nutrient-rich breakfast with sweet potato hash. Dice sweet potatoes and cook them in a skillet with diced bacon or sausage, onions, and garlic until golden brown and crispy. Add in chopped kale or spinach and cook until wilted. Serve topped with fried eggs and a drizzle of hot sauce for extra flavor.

Lunch Recipes:

Grilled Chicken Salad: Prepare a refreshing and satisfying salad with grilled chicken breast, mixed greens, cherry tomatoes, cucumber slices, avocado chunks, and sliced almonds. Dress the salad with a simple vinaigrette made with olive oil, balsamic vinegar, Dijon mustard, and fresh herbs.

Salmon Nori Wraps: Create a portable and nutritious lunch with salmon nori wraps. Lay a sheet of nori on a flat surface and spread mashed avocado over the surface. Top with cooked salmon fillet, thinly sliced cucumber, and shredded carrots. Roll up the nori tightly and slice into bite-sized pieces for a delicious and satisfying meal.

Dinner Recipes:

Bison and Vegetable Stir-Fry: Prepare a flavorful stir-fry using lean bison meat and an assortment of colorful vegetables. Slice bison meat thinly and stir-fry in a hot skillet with sliced onions, bell peppers, broccoli florets, and snap peas. Season with coconut aminos, garlic, ginger, and red pepper flakes for a delicious and savory dish.

Zucchini Noodle Bolognese: Enjoy a lighter take on a classic Italian dish with zucchini noodle bolognese. Spiralize zucchini into noodles and sauté in a skillet with olive oil until tender. Meanwhile, prepare a hearty bolognese sauce with ground grass-fed beef, diced tomatoes, tomato paste, garlic, onions, and Italian herbs. Serve the bolognese sauce over the zucchini noodles and garnish with fresh basil and grated Parmesan cheese.

Snack Recipes:

Trail Mix: Prepare a homemade trail mix using a variety of nuts, seeds, and dried fruits. Mix together almonds, walnuts, pumpkin seeds, sunflower seeds, and dried cranberries or raisins for a delicious and nutrient-rich snack. Portion the trail mix into individual snack bags for convenient grab-and-go snacking.

Roasted Vegetable Chips: Make crispy and flavorful vegetable chips by thinly slicing vegetables such as sweet potatoes, beets, and kale. Toss the sliced vegetables with olive oil, sea salt, and your favorite spices, then spread them out in a single layer on a baking sheet. Bake in the oven at a low temperature until crispy and golden brown for a nutritious and satisfying snack.

Conclusion:

These breakfast, lunch, dinner, and snack recipes inspired by our ancestors offer a delicious and nutritious way to embrace ancestral eating principles. By prioritizing whole, minimally processed ingredients and incorporating a variety of nutrient-dense foods, these recipes provide nourishment for the body and support overall health and well-being. Whether you're looking for a hearty breakfast, a satisfying lunch, a flavorful dinner, or a nutritious snack, these recipes offer something for every meal of the day. Enjoy the flavors and benefits of ancestral eating with these delicious and satisfying recipes.

Traditional dishes from different cultures

Traditional dishes from different cultures offer a rich tapestry of flavors, textures, and culinary traditions that reflect the unique heritage and history of each region. From hearty stews and savory curries to delicate pastries and sweet desserts, traditional dishes showcase the diversity and creativity of global cuisine. In this exploration of traditional dishes from different cultures, we'll journey around the world to discover iconic recipes that have been passed down through generations, preserving cultural identity and culinary heritage.

1. Italian Cuisine:

Pasta Carbonara: Originating from Rome, pasta carbonara is a classic Italian dish made with pasta, eggs, pancetta or guanciale (cured pork jowl), Parmesan cheese, and black pepper. The dish is known for its creamy texture and rich flavor, with the eggs and cheese creating a luxurious sauce that coats the pasta. Pasta carbonara is a comforting and satisfying dish that showcases the simplicity and elegance of Italian cuisine.

2. Mexican Cuisine:

Tacos al Pastor: Tacos al pastor is a popular street food dish in Mexico, particularly in Mexico City. It features marinated pork that is thinly sliced and stacked on a vertical rotisserie, similar to shawarma. The pork is typically seasoned with a blend of spices, including achiote, garlic, and citrus juices, then roasted until tender and flavorful. The sliced pork is served on small corn tortillas and topped with pineapple, onions, cilantro, and salsa for a burst of sweet, savory, and spicy flavors.

3. Indian Cuisine:

Chicken Tikka Masala: Chicken tikka masala is a beloved Indian dish that has gained popularity worldwide. It consists of marinated chicken pieces that are grilled and then simmered in a creamy tomato-based sauce spiced with garam masala, turmeric, cumin, and other aromatic spices. The sauce is rich and flavorful, with a balance of tangy, sweet, and savory notes. Chicken tikka masala is typically served with rice or naan bread for a hearty and satisfying meal.

4. Chinese Cuisine:

Mapo Tofu: Mapo tofu is a spicy and flavorful dish from the Sichuan province of China. It features silken tofu cooked in a spicy sauce made with fermented black beans, chili paste, garlic, and Sichuan peppercorns. Ground pork or beef is often added to the sauce for extra flavor and texture. Mapo tofu is known for its numbing and spicy flavor profile, making it a favorite among fans of Sichuan cuisine.

5. French Cuisine:

Coq au Vin: Coq au vin is a classic French dish that originated in the Burgundy region of France. It features chicken braised in red wine with mushrooms, onions, bacon, and garlic. The dish is slow-cooked until the chicken is tender and infused with the rich flavors of the wine and aromatics. Coq au vin is typically served with crusty bread or mashed potatoes for a comforting and hearty meal.

6. Japanese Cuisine:

Sushi: Sushi is a traditional Japanese dish that has become popular worldwide. It consists of vinegared rice served with a variety of toppings, including raw or cooked seafood, vegetables, and occasionally tropical fruits. The most well-known type of sushi is nigiri, which consists of a small mound of rice topped with a slice of fish or seafood. Other popular types of sushi include maki (rolled sushi) and sashimi (sliced raw fish).

7. Greek Cuisine:

Moussaka: Moussaka is a classic Greek dish made with layers of eggplant, ground meat (usually lamb or beef), and a creamy béchamel sauce. The dish is seasoned with aromatic spices such as cinnamon, nutmeg, and oregano, giving it a rich and flavorful taste. Moussaka is typically baked until golden and bubbly, then served warm as a hearty and comforting meal.

8. Thai Cuisine:

Tom Yum Goong: Tom yum goong is a spicy and sour soup from Thailand that features shrimp as the main ingredient. The soup is flavored with lemongrass, kaffir lime leaves, galangal, fish sauce, and chili peppers, giving it a bold and aromatic flavor profile. Additional ingredients such as mushrooms, tomatoes, and herbs are often added to enhance the complexity of the soup. Tom yum goong is typically served hot as a starter or main course in Thai cuisine.

9. Spanish Cuisine:

Paella: Paella is a traditional Spanish rice dish that originated in the Valencia region of Spain. It features a flavorful combination of rice, saffron, seafood, meat (such as chicken or rabbit), and vegetables. The dish is cooked in a wide, shallow pan called a paellera, which allows the rice to develop a crispy crust on the bottom known as socarrat. Paella is often served as a communal dish, with diners sharing from the same pan.

10. Lebanese Cuisine:

Hummus: Hummus is a popular Middle Eastern dip made from cooked chickpeas, tahini (sesame paste), garlic, lemon juice, and olive oil. The ingredients are blended together until smooth and creamy, resulting in a delicious and nutritious dip that is often served with pita bread or fresh vegetables. Hummus is a staple in Lebanese cuisine and is enjoyed as a snack, appetizer, or accompaniment to meals.

In conclusion, traditional dishes from different cultures offer a diverse and flavorful culinary experience that reflects the unique heritage and culinary traditions of each region. From hearty stews and savory curries to delicate pastries and sweet desserts, these dishes showcase the creativity, complexity, and richness of global cuisine. Whether you're craving the comforting flavors of Italian pasta carbonara, the bold spices of Indian chicken tikka masala, or the fresh and vibrant ingredients of Mexican tacos al pastor, traditional dishes from different cultures invite you to embark on a delicious journey around the world.

Tips for sourcing quality ingredients

Sourcing quality ingredients is essential for creating delicious and nutritious meals that showcase the best flavors and textures. Whether you're shopping for fresh produce, meat, seafood, grains, or pantry staples, selecting high-quality ingredients can elevate your cooking and enhance the overall dining experience. In this guide, we'll explore tips for sourcing quality ingredients to help you make informed decisions and support your culinary endeavors.

1. Shop Seasonally:
One of the best ways to ensure quality ingredients is to shop seasonally. Seasonal produce is typically fresher, tastier, and more affordable since it's harvested at its peak ripeness and doesn't need to be transported long distances. Visit your local farmers' market or join a community-supported agriculture (CSA) program to access a wide variety of seasonal fruits and vegetables that are grown locally and sustainably.

2. Know Your Suppliers:
Establishing relationships with trusted suppliers is key to sourcing quality ingredients. Whether you're shopping at a farmers' market, specialty grocery store, or online retailer, take the time to learn about the sourcing practices and standards of the suppliers you're purchasing from. Look for suppliers who prioritize organic, sustainable, and ethically sourced ingredients and are transparent about their farming and production methods.

3. Choose Organic Whenever Possible:
Opting for organic ingredients can help ensure that you're getting high-quality produce and products that are free from synthetic pesticides, herbicides, and genetically modified organisms (GMOs). Look for the USDA Organic or equivalent certification on packaged products and inquire about organic options when shopping for fresh produce and meat.

4. Read Labels Carefully:
When purchasing packaged or processed foods, reading labels carefully is essential for sourcing quality ingredients. Look for products with simple, recognizable ingredients and avoid those that contain artificial additives, preservatives, and high levels of refined sugars, sodium, or unhealthy fats. Choose products with minimal processing and ingredients that you can pronounce and understand.

5. Consider Local and Artisanal Options:
Supporting local and artisanal producers is a great way to source quality ingredients while also contributing to your community's economy and food system. Look for locally produced fruits, vegetables, dairy products, meats, and artisanal goods such as bread, cheese, and preserves at farmers' markets, independent grocery stores, and specialty food shops.

6. Explore Specialty Stores and Markets:
Specialty stores and markets are excellent sources for finding unique and high-quality ingredients that may be difficult to find elsewhere. Explore specialty grocers, ethnic markets, butcher shops, fishmongers, and gourmet food stores in your area to discover a wide range of specialty ingredients, imported goods, and artisanal products.

7. Prioritize Freshness:
When shopping for fresh produce, meat, seafood, and dairy products, prioritize freshness to ensure optimal quality and flavor. Look for fruits and vegetables that are firm, vibrant in color, and free from bruises or blemishes. Choose meats and seafood that are fresh, properly stored, and sourced from reputable suppliers. When possible, select products with the shortest shelf life to ensure maximum freshness.

8. Consider Sustainability:
Choosing sustainable ingredients is not only good for the environment but also ensures that you're supporting responsible farming and fishing practices. Look for certifications such as the Marine Stewardship Council (MSC) for seafood and the Rainforest Alliance for coffee, tea, and chocolate to identify sustainably sourced products. Consider factors such as environmental impact, animal welfare, and social responsibility when sourcing ingredients.

9. Shop at Whole Foods Markets:
Whole Foods Markets are known for their commitment to quality and selection of organic, natural, and responsibly sourced ingredients. With a focus on transparency and sustainability, Whole Foods offers a wide range of high-quality produce, meats, seafood, dairy products, and pantry staples that meet rigorous quality standards. Shop at Whole Foods Markets for a diverse selection of quality ingredients and specialty products.

10. Support Farmer's Markets:
Farmer's markets are excellent sources for sourcing quality ingredients directly from local farmers and producers. By shopping at farmer's markets, you can access fresh, seasonal produce, meats, dairy products, and artisanal goods that are grown and produced locally and sustainably. Connect with farmers and producers, ask questions about their farming practices, and learn about the origin of the ingredients you're purchasing.

11. Use Online Resources:
Online resources such as specialty food websites, farmer's market directories, and online retailers offer convenient ways to source quality ingredients from the comfort of your home. Explore online platforms that specialize in organic, natural, and artisanal products, and consider subscribing to delivery services that offer fresh produce boxes, meat and seafood subscriptions, and specialty ingredient kits.

12. Consider Food Safety:
When sourcing ingredients, it's important to consider food safety and ensure that the products you're purchasing meet strict quality and safety standards. Look for products that are labeled with certifications such as USDA Organic, Non-GMO Project Verified, and GFSI (Global Food Safety Initiative) certifications. Follow proper food handling and storage practices to maintain the quality and safety of your ingredients.

Conclusion:
Sourcing quality ingredients is essential for creating delicious, nutritious, and memorable meals that highlight the best flavors and textures. By shopping seasonally, knowing your suppliers, choosing organic whenever possible, reading labels carefully, considering local and artisanal options, exploring specialty stores and markets, prioritizing freshness, considering sustainability, shopping at Whole Foods Markets, supporting farmer's markets, using online resources, and considering food safety, you can make informed decisions and source high-quality ingredients for your culinary endeavors. Whether you're cooking at home or dining out, sourcing quality ingredients ensures that you're enjoying the best flavors and nutritional benefits that food has to offer.

Chapter 8

Navigating Modern Challenges

Navigating modern challenges such as eating out and social situations can be daunting, especially when trying to maintain a healthy and balanced diet. Whether you're dining at restaurants, attending social gatherings, or traveling, it's important to have strategies in place to make informed choices and stay on track with your dietary goals. In this guide, we'll explore tips and strategies for navigating eating out and social situations while prioritizing health and well-being.

Eating Out:

Research Restaurants in Advance:
Before dining out, take the time to research restaurants in your area that offer healthy and nutritious options. Look for restaurants that prioritize fresh, locally sourced ingredients and offer a variety of dishes that align with your dietary preferences and restrictions. Many restaurants now provide menus online, allowing you to review options and make informed choices before arriving.

Choose Restaurants with Healthy Options:
Select restaurants that offer a diverse selection of healthy and nutritious options, including salads, grilled proteins, vegetable-based dishes, and whole grain options. Avoid restaurants known for their heavy, fried, or overly processed menu items, and opt for establishments that focus on fresh, wholesome ingredients prepared in a health-conscious manner.

Customize Your Order:
Don't hesitate to customize your order to suit your dietary preferences and restrictions. Ask for substitutions or modifications to dishes to accommodate your needs, such as swapping out fries for a side salad or requesting sauces and dressings on the side. Most restaurants are willing to accommodate dietary requests within reason, so don't be afraid to ask.

Portion Control:
Pay attention to portion sizes when dining out, as restaurant servings are often larger than what you would typically eat at home. Consider sharing entrees with dining companions or asking for a half portion if available. Alternatively, ask for a to-go box when your meal is served and portion out a smaller serving to enjoy at the restaurant, saving the rest for later.

Mindful Eating:
Practice mindful eating when dining out by paying attention to hunger cues, eating slowly, and savoring each bite. Focus on the flavors, textures, and aromas of your food, and listen to your body's signals of fullness to prevent overeating. Avoid distractions such as electronic devices and engage in conversation with dining companions to enhance the dining experience.

Watch for Hidden Calories:
Be mindful of hidden calories in restaurant dishes, particularly in sauces, dressings, and condiments. Opt for lighter options such as vinaigrettes or olive oil-based dressings instead of creamy or high-fat sauces. Ask for sauces and dressings on the side so you can control the amount you consume.

Social Situations:

Communicate Your Dietary Needs:
When attending social gatherings or events, communicate your dietary needs and restrictions to the host or organizer in advance. Offer to bring a dish or snack that aligns with your dietary preferences, ensuring that you have a healthy option to enjoy.

Plan Ahead:
If you know you'll be attending a social event where unhealthy food choices may be prevalent, plan ahead by eating a balanced meal or snack beforehand. This can help curb hunger and prevent overindulgence in less healthy options at the event.

Be Selective:
Be selective about your food choices when faced with a variety of options at social gatherings. Scan the food spread and prioritize healthier options such as fresh fruits, vegetables, lean proteins, and whole grains. Allow yourself to indulge in small portions of your favorite treats while balancing them with nutrient-dense options.

Stay Hydrated:
Stay hydrated throughout social gatherings by drinking water or other non-caloric beverages. This can help prevent mindless snacking and keep you feeling full and satisfied. Avoid sugary drinks and alcoholic beverages, which can contribute to excess calorie intake.

Practice Moderation:
Practice moderation when indulging in treats and desserts at social events. Allow yourself to enjoy small portions of your favorite treats without feeling guilty or deprived. Focus on savoring the flavors and enjoying the experience without overindulging.

Engage in Activities:
Engage in activities and conversations at social gatherings to distract yourself from mindless snacking and grazing. Participate in games, take a walk, or engage in meaningful conversations with friends and family to stay active and present during the event.

Be Mindful of Alcohol Intake:
Be mindful of your alcohol intake at social gatherings, as alcoholic beverages can contribute to excess calorie consumption and impair judgment around food choices. Opt for lighter options such as wine spritzers or low-calorie cocktails, and alternate alcoholic drinks with water to stay hydrated.

Conclusion:

Navigating modern challenges such as eating out and social situations requires thoughtful planning, communication, and mindfulness. By researching restaurants in advance, choosing healthy options, customizing your order, practicing portion control, and staying mindful of hidden calories when dining out, you can make informed choices that align with your dietary goals. Similarly, communicating your dietary needs, planning ahead, being selective about food choices, staying hydrated, practicing moderation, and engaging in activities during social gatherings can help you navigate social situations while prioritizing health and well-being. With these tips and strategies in mind, you can confidently navigate eating out and social situations while maintaining a balanced and healthy lifestyle.

Dealing with cravings and temptations

Dealing with cravings and temptations is a common challenge that many people face when trying to maintain a healthy and balanced diet. Whether it's the allure of sugary treats, salty snacks, or indulgent desserts, cravings can often derail even the most well-intentioned dietary plans. However, with the right strategies and mindset, it's possible to manage cravings and resist temptations while still enjoying a satisfying and nourishing diet. In this guide, we'll explore tips and techniques for dealing with cravings and temptations to help you stay on track with your health and wellness goals.

Understanding Cravings:

Before diving into strategies for managing cravings, it's important to understand what causes them in the first place. Cravings can be triggered by a variety of factors, including physiological, psychological, and environmental cues. Physiologically, cravings may arise due to fluctuations in blood sugar levels, hormonal imbalances, or nutrient deficiencies. Psychologically, cravings may be linked to emotional triggers such as stress, boredom, or anxiety. Additionally, environmental factors such as exposure to food advertisements, social influences, and cultural norms can also influence cravings.

Strategies for Dealing with Cravings:

Identify Triggers: Start by identifying your specific triggers for cravings. Keep a food diary to track when cravings occur, what foods you crave, and any patterns or trends that emerge. This can help you identify underlying factors that may be contributing to your cravings, such as emotional triggers, hormonal fluctuations, or environmental cues.

Address Underlying Needs: Once you've identified your triggers, work on addressing the underlying needs that may be driving your cravings. For example, if you tend to crave sugary foods when stressed, explore alternative stress-relief strategies such as meditation, exercise, or spending time outdoors. If you crave salty snacks when bored, find engaging activities or hobbies to keep yourself occupied.

Practice Mindful Eating: Incorporate mindfulness into your eating habits to help manage cravings and resist temptations. Pay attention to hunger and fullness cues, eat slowly, and savor each bite of food. Be present and mindful during meals, focusing on the sensory experience of eating and enjoying the flavors, textures, and aromas of your food.

Stay Hydrated: Dehydration can sometimes masquerade as hunger or cravings, leading you to reach for food when you're actually thirsty. Stay hydrated throughout the day by drinking plenty of water and other non-caloric beverages. Keep a water bottle with you and sip on water regularly to prevent dehydration and reduce cravings.

Eat Balanced Meals: Prioritize balanced meals that include a combination of protein, fiber, healthy fats, and complex carbohydrates to help stabilize blood sugar levels and prevent cravings. Include lean proteins such as poultry, fish, tofu, or legumes, along with plenty of vegetables, whole grains, and healthy fats from sources like avocado, nuts, and olive oil.

Include Regular Snacks: Incorporate regular, balanced snacks into your day to help prevent extreme hunger and cravings between meals. Choose nutrient-dense snacks such as Greek yogurt with berries, apple slices with almond butter, or vegetable sticks with hummus to keep you satisfied and energized throughout the day.

Plan Ahead: Anticipate and plan for cravings by having healthy, satisfying alternatives on hand. Stock your pantry and fridge with nutritious snacks and ingredients that you enjoy, so you have options readily available when cravings strike. Pre-portion snacks into individual servings to prevent overeating and mindless snacking.

Practice Moderation: Allow yourself to indulge in small portions of your favorite treats occasionally, rather than completely restricting them. Depriving yourself of foods you enjoy can sometimes backfire and lead to intensified cravings and overeating. Practice moderation and mindfulness when enjoying treats, savoring each bite and enjoying the experience without guilt or judgment.

Distract Yourself: When cravings strike, distract yourself with activities or tasks that can help shift your focus away from food. Engage in hobbies, go for a walk, call a friend, or tackle a project to occupy your mind and redirect your attention. By engaging in activities that bring you joy and fulfillment, you can reduce the intensity of cravings and resist temptations more effectively.

Seek Support: Don't hesitate to reach out for support from friends, family, or a healthcare professional if you're struggling to manage cravings on your own. Share your challenges and experiences with others who can offer encouragement, accountability, and practical advice. Consider joining a support group or seeking guidance from a registered dietitian or therapist who specializes in mindful eating and behavior change.

Conclusion:

Dealing with cravings and temptations is a common challenge that many people face when trying to maintain a healthy and balanced diet. By understanding the underlying causes of cravings, addressing your specific triggers, practicing mindful eating, staying hydrated, eating balanced meals, including regular snacks, planning ahead, practicing moderation, distracting yourself, and seeking support when needed, you can effectively manage cravings and resist temptations while still enjoying a satisfying and nourishing diet. With patience, practice, and perseverance, you can develop healthy habits and strategies to navigate cravings and stay on track with your health and wellness goals.

Staying motivated and committed

Staying motivated and committed to your health and wellness goals is essential for long-term success and sustainability. Whether you're striving to eat healthier, exercise regularly, manage stress, or achieve other lifestyle changes, maintaining motivation and commitment can be challenging, especially when faced with obstacles and setbacks. In this guide, we'll explore strategies and techniques for staying motivated and committed to your health and wellness journey.

1. Set Clear and Realistic Goals:
Start by setting clear, specific, and achievable goals that align with your values and priorities. Break down larger goals into smaller, manageable steps, and set realistic timelines for achieving them. Having clear goals gives you a sense of direction and purpose, motivating you to stay focused and committed to your health and wellness journey.

2. Find Your Why:
Identify your reasons for wanting to make positive changes in your life and connect with your deeper motivations. Reflect on how achieving your health and wellness goals will improve your quality of life, enhance your well-being, and align with your values and aspirations. Understanding your "why" can provide a powerful source of motivation and inspiration during challenging times.

3. Celebrate Progress:
Celebrate your progress and accomplishments along the way, no matter how small they may seem. Acknowledge and celebrate each milestone, whether it's reaching a fitness goal, making healthier food choices, or practicing self-care. Celebrating progress reinforces positive behaviors and motivates you to continue moving forward on your health and wellness journey.

4. Create a Supportive Environment:
Surround yourself with a supportive environment that encourages and reinforces your health and wellness goals. Build a support network of friends, family members, or peers who share similar goals and can provide encouragement, accountability, and practical support. Engage in activities and environments that align with your goals and values, minimizing exposure to negative influences or temptations.

5. Practice Self-Compassion:
Be kind to yourself and practice self-compassion as you navigate your health and wellness journey. Accept that setbacks and challenges are a natural part of the process and treat yourself with kindness and understanding during difficult times. Instead of dwelling on mistakes or perceived failures, focus on learning from them and moving forward with renewed determination.

6. Stay Flexible and Adapt:
Stay flexible and adaptable in your approach to health and wellness, recognizing that your journey may involve detours and adjustments along the way. Be open to trying new strategies, experimenting with different approaches, and adapting your goals and plans as needed based on feedback and results. Embrace a growth mindset that views challenges as opportunities for growth and learning.

7. Find Meaning and Purpose:
Connect your health and wellness goals to a deeper sense of meaning and purpose in your life. Consider how prioritizing your health and well-being aligns with your values, passions, and long-term aspirations. Cultivate a sense of purpose and fulfillment by focusing on activities and behaviors that bring you joy, satisfaction, and fulfillment.

8. Practice Self-Care:
Prioritize self-care practices that nourish your body, mind, and spirit and support your overall well-being. Make time for activities that rejuvenate and energize you, such as exercise, meditation, hobbies, or spending time in nature. Take care of your physical, emotional, and mental health by prioritizing sleep, managing stress, and seeking support when needed.

9. Stay Inspired and Educated:
Stay inspired and educated by seeking out sources of inspiration, motivation, and knowledge related to health and wellness. Surround yourself with positive influences such as books, podcasts, blogs, or social media accounts that align with your goals and values. Stay informed about the latest research, trends, and best practices in health and wellness to empower yourself with knowledge and motivation.

10. Focus on the Journey, Not Just the Destination:
Shift your focus from solely achieving outcomes to embracing the journey of personal growth and self-discovery. Embrace the process of learning, growing, and evolving as you work towards your health and wellness goals. Celebrate the daily habits, practices, and behaviors that contribute to your overall well-being, recognizing that true success lies in the journey itself.

Conclusion:

Staying motivated and committed to your health and wellness goals requires dedication, perseverance, and self-awareness. By setting clear and realistic goals, finding your why, celebrating progress, creating a supportive environment, practicing self-compassion, staying flexible and adaptable, finding meaning and purpose, prioritizing self-care, staying inspired and educated, and focusing on the journey, you can maintain motivation and commitment on your health and wellness journey. Remember that progress is not always linear, and setbacks are a natural part of the process. Stay patient, stay persistent, and stay committed to your health and well-being, knowing that every step forward brings you closer to achieving your goals and living your best life.

Chapter 9

Success Stories: Real-Life Experiences with Ancestral Eating

Raymond's Success Story with Ancestral Eating:

Raymond had struggled with weight management and chronic health issues for most of his adult life. Despite trying various diets and exercise programs, he found it challenging to maintain a healthy weight and experienced frequent fluctuations in his energy levels and overall well-being. Frustrated with the lack of sustainable results, Raymond began researching alternative approaches to nutrition and stumbled upon the concept of ancestral eating.

Intrigued by the idea of returning to a diet based on the foods our ancestors consumed, Raymond decided to give ancestral eating a try. He started by incorporating more whole, unprocessed foods into his diet, including lean proteins, fresh fruits and vegetables, nuts, seeds, and healthy fats. He focused on sourcing high-quality, nutrient-dense ingredients and prioritized organic, grass-fed, and locally sourced options whenever possible.

As Raymond began to adopt the principles of ancestral eating, he noticed significant improvements in his health and well-being. He experienced increased energy levels, improved mental clarity, and better digestion. He also noticed that his cravings for processed foods and sugary snacks diminished, and he felt more satisfied and satiated after meals.

Over time, Raymond's commitment to ancestral eating paid off in tangible ways. He achieved a healthier weight, shedding excess pounds without feeling deprived or restricted. His blood sugar levels stabilized, and he experienced fewer cravings and mood swings throughout the day. Raymond also noticed improvements in his athletic performance and recovery time, allowing him to engage in regular exercise with greater ease and enjoyment.

Beyond the physical benefits, Raymond found that ancestral eating had a profound impact on his overall quality of life. He felt more connected to his food and the natural world, appreciating the simplicity and nourishment of whole, unprocessed foods. He enjoyed exploring new recipes and cooking techniques inspired by ancestral traditions, finding joy and satisfaction in preparing meals from scratch.

Today, Raymond continues to embrace ancestral eating as a sustainable and fulfilling way of nourishing his body and supporting his health and well-being. He feels grateful for the positive changes he has experienced and is committed to sharing his success story with others who may be seeking a similar path to improved health through ancestral eating.

Salomey's Success Story with Ancestral Eating

Salomey had always been interested in health and nutrition, but she struggled to find a diet that worked for her unique needs and preferences. She experimented with various eating styles, from veganism to low-carb diets, but none provided the sustainable results she desired. Frustrated and feeling discouraged, Salomey was determined to find a more balanced and holistic approach to eating.

Upon discovering the principles of ancestral eating, Salomey was intrigued by the idea of returning to a diet based on whole, unprocessed foods that our ancestors would have consumed. She appreciated the focus on nutrient density and quality, as well as the emphasis on incorporating a variety of foods from nature's bounty. Excited to embark on a new culinary journey, Salomey embraced ancestral eating with enthusiasm.

Salomey started by incorporating more whole foods into her diet, including grass-fed meats, wild-caught fish, organic fruits and vegetables, nuts, seeds, and healthy fats like avocado and olive oil. She prioritized nutrient-dense foods and avoided processed and refined products as much as possible. Salomey also experimented with traditional cooking methods and recipes inspired by ancestral cuisines from around the world.

As Salomey transitioned to an ancestral eating lifestyle, she began to experience significant improvements in her health and well-being. She noticed that her energy levels stabilized, and she felt more sustained throughout the day. Salomey also found that her digestion improved, and she experienced fewer digestive issues and bloating after meals.

One of the most profound changes Salomey noticed was in her mental clarity and cognitive function. She felt sharper and more focused, with improved concentration and memory. Salomey also experienced better mood regulation and emotional balance, attributing these changes to the nourishing and balanced nature of her ancestral eating diet.

Over time, Salomey's commitment to ancestral eating paid off in numerous ways. She achieved a healthy weight and body composition without feeling deprived or restricted. Her skin became clearer, and she noticed an overall improvement in her complexion and skin tone. Salomey also found that she slept better and woke up feeling more refreshed and rejuvenated each morning.

Beyond the physical and mental benefits, Salomey found that ancestral eating had a profound impact on her overall lifestyle and well-being. She felt more connected to her food and the natural world, appreciating the simplicity and purity of whole, unprocessed ingredients. Salomey also enjoyed the sense of community and camaraderie that came with exploring ancestral cooking techniques and recipes with like-minded individuals.

Today, Salomey continues to embrace ancestral eating as a sustainable and fulfilling way of nourishing her body and supporting her health and well-being. She feels empowered by her success with ancestral eating and is committed to sharing her journey and inspiring others to explore the transformative power of whole, unprocessed foods and ancestral cooking traditions.

Overcoming Health Challenges Through Ancestral Eating:

Ancestral eating, which focuses on consuming whole, unprocessed foods similar to what our ancestors ate, has gained popularity for its potential to address various health challenges. Many individuals have experienced significant improvements in their health and well-being by adopting ancestral eating principles. Let's explore some common health challenges and how ancestral eating can help overcome them:

Weight Management: Ancestral eating emphasizes nutrient-dense foods such as lean proteins, fruits, vegetables, and healthy fats while minimizing processed and refined foods. This approach can support weight management by promoting satiety, stabilizing blood sugar levels, and reducing cravings for unhealthy foods. By focusing on whole, nutrient-rich foods, individuals can achieve and maintain a healthy weight more effectively.

Digestive Issues: Many people experience digestive issues such as bloating, gas, and discomfort due to modern diets high in processed foods, additives, and artificial ingredients. Ancestral eating emphasizes whole, unprocessed foods that are easier to digest and less likely to cause gastrointestinal distress. By prioritizing fiber-rich fruits and vegetables, probiotic-rich fermented foods, and gut-friendly fats, individuals can support digestive health and alleviate symptoms of digestive issues.

Blood Sugar Regulation: Ancestral eating promotes a balanced intake of macronutrients, including proteins, fats, and carbohydrates, which can help regulate blood sugar levels and prevent spikes and crashes. By prioritizing complex carbohydrates from fruits, vegetables, and whole grains, along with healthy fats and proteins, individuals can support stable blood sugar levels and reduce the risk of insulin resistance and type 2 diabetes.

Heart Health: Ancestral eating emphasizes heart-healthy fats such as those found in nuts, seeds, avocados, and fatty fish, which can help improve cholesterol levels and reduce the risk of heart disease. By prioritizing these healthy fats and minimizing intake of processed and trans fats, individuals can support heart health and reduce the risk of cardiovascular issues.

Inflammation: Chronic inflammation is linked to many health conditions, including autoimmune diseases, arthritis, and metabolic syndrome. Ancestral eating emphasizes anti-inflammatory foods such as fruits, vegetables, nuts, seeds, and fatty fish, while minimizing pro-inflammatory processed foods and refined sugars. By adopting an anti-inflammatory diet rich in whole, nutrient-dense foods, individuals can reduce inflammation levels and support overall health and well-being.

Energy Levels and Mental Clarity: Ancestral eating focuses on whole, nutrient-dense foods that provide sustained energy and support cognitive function. By prioritizing foods rich in vitamins, minerals, and antioxidants, individuals can improve energy levels, mental clarity, and focus. Additionally, avoiding processed foods and refined sugars can prevent energy crashes and brain fog, leading to improved cognitive function and overall well-being.

Immune Function: Ancestral eating emphasizes foods that support immune function, such as fruits, vegetables, herbs, and spices rich in vitamins, minerals, and antioxidants. By prioritizing these immune-boosting foods and minimizing intake of processed foods and added sugars that can weaken immune function, individuals can support a strong and resilient immune system.

Overall, ancestral eating offers a holistic approach to nutrition that can help individuals overcome a variety of health challenges by focusing on whole, unprocessed foods that nourish the body and support optimal health and well-being. By prioritizing nutrient-dense foods and minimizing processed and refined foods, individuals can experience significant improvements in their health, vitality, and overall quality of life.

Chapter 10

Conclusion: Embracing a Healthier Future

Key Takeaways from Ancestral Eating:

Ancestral eating, also known as the paleo or primal diet, is a dietary approach based on the types of foods our ancestors would have eaten during the Paleolithic era. This approach emphasizes whole, unprocessed foods such as lean proteins, fruits, vegetables, nuts, seeds, and healthy fats while avoiding processed and refined foods, grains, legumes, and dairy products. By focusing on nutrient-dense, whole foods that are closer to what our ancestors would have consumed, ancestral eating aims to promote optimal health, support weight management, improve digestion, regulate blood sugar levels, and reduce inflammation.

1. Emphasize Whole, Unprocessed Foods:
Ancestral eating prioritizes whole, unprocessed foods that are rich in nutrients and free from additives, preservatives, and artificial ingredients. This includes lean proteins such as grass-fed meats, wild-caught fish, and free-range poultry, as well as a variety of fruits, vegetables, nuts, seeds, and healthy fats like avocado, olive oil, and coconut oil.

2. Minimize Processed and Refined Foods:
Ancestral eating avoids processed and refined foods such as sugary snacks, processed meats, refined grains, and vegetable oils that are commonly found in modern diets. These foods are often low in nutrients and can contribute to weight gain, inflammation, and various health issues when consumed in excess.

3. Prioritize Nutrient Density:
Ancestral eating focuses on nutrient-dense foods that provide a wide range of vitamins, minerals, antioxidants, and phytonutrients essential for optimal health and well-being. By prioritizing nutrient-dense foods such as fruits, vegetables, nuts, seeds, and lean proteins, individuals can ensure they are meeting their nutritional needs and supporting overall health.

4. Support Sustainable and Ethical Food Choices:
Ancestral eating encourages sustainable and ethical food choices, including sourcing grass-fed meats, wild-caught fish, organic fruits and vegetables, and pasture-raised eggs whenever possible. By supporting sustainable farming and fishing practices, individuals can minimize their environmental impact and promote animal welfare.

5. Focus on Quality Over Quantity:
Ancestral eating emphasizes quality over quantity when it comes to food choices. Instead of focusing solely on calorie counting or strict portion control, individuals are encouraged to prioritize the quality of their food by choosing nutrient-dense, whole foods that nourish the body and support optimal health.

6. Listen to Your Body:
Ancestral eating encourages individuals to listen to their bodies and pay attention to hunger and fullness cues. By practicing mindful eating and tuning into their body's signals, individuals can better regulate their food intake and make choices that support their nutritional needs and overall well-being.

7. Experiment and Adapt:
Ancestral eating is not a one-size-fits-all approach, and individuals are encouraged to experiment with different foods and eating patterns to find what works best for their unique needs and preferences. This may involve adapting the diet to accommodate food sensitivities, allergies, or specific health goals.

8. Focus on Long-Term Health and Well-Being:
Ancestral eating emphasizes a holistic approach to health and well-being that goes beyond short-term weight loss or dietary restrictions. By focusing on whole, unprocessed foods that support optimal health and vitality, individuals can experience long-term benefits such as improved energy levels, better digestion, reduced inflammation, and enhanced overall well-being.

9. Seek Balance and Enjoyment:
Ancestral eating encourages individuals to seek balance and enjoyment in their food choices and dietary habits. While prioritizing nutrient-dense, whole foods is important, individuals are also encouraged to indulge in occasional treats and enjoy the social and cultural aspects of eating without guilt or restriction.

10. Stay Informed and Open-Minded:
Ancestral eating is a dynamic and evolving approach to nutrition, and individuals are encouraged to stay informed about the latest research, trends, and best practices in the field. By remaining open-minded and willing to adapt their dietary habits based on new information and personal experiences, individuals can continue to optimize their health and well-being through ancestral eating.

Overall, ancestral eating offers a holistic and sustainable approach to nutrition that prioritizes whole, unprocessed foods, supports optimal health and well-being, and encourages individuals to listen to their bodies and make choices that align with their unique needs and preferences. By embracing the principles of ancestral eating and incorporating nutrient-dense, whole foods into their diets, individuals can experience a wide range of health benefits and improve their overall quality of life.

Encouragement for Continuing the Journey with Ancestral Eating:

Embarking on a journey towards better health and well-being through ancestral eating is a courageous and empowering decision. As you navigate this path, it's important to acknowledge that change takes time and effort, and there may be challenges along the way. However, the rewards of prioritizing whole, unprocessed foods and nourishing your body with nutrient-dense ingredients are well worth the journey. Here are some words of encouragement to inspire you to continue your journey with ancestral eating:

1. Celebrate Your Progress: Take a moment to celebrate how far you've come on your journey with ancestral eating. Whether you've made small changes to your diet or fully embraced the principles of ancestral eating, every step forward is a victory worth celebrating. Acknowledge the positive changes you've experienced in your health, energy levels, and overall well-being, and use them as motivation to keep moving forward.

2. Embrace Imperfection: Remember that nobody's journey with ancestral eating is perfect, and that's okay. There may be days when you veer off course or indulge in foods that don't align with ancestral eating principles, and that's part of being human. Instead of dwelling on setbacks or perceived failures, embrace imperfection as an opportunity for growth and learning. Be kind to yourself, practice self-compassion, and use setbacks as motivation to recommit to your health and well-being goals.

3. Focus on the Long-Term Benefits: Keep your eyes on the prize and focus on the long-term benefits of ancestral eating. While it's easy to get caught up in short-term results or setbacks, remember that true health and well-being are a journey, not a destination. By prioritizing whole, unprocessed foods and nourishing your body with nutrient-dense ingredients, you are investing in your long-term health and vitality. Keep reminding yourself of the positive impact ancestral eating can have on your overall quality of life, and let that motivate you to stay the course.

4. Cultivate Resilience: As you continue your journey with ancestral eating, cultivate resilience and perseverance in the face of challenges. There may be times when you encounter obstacles or setbacks, whether it's navigating social situations, dealing with cravings, or facing criticism from others. In these moments, draw upon your inner strength and resilience to stay true to your health and well-being goals. Remember that setbacks are temporary, and every challenge you overcome makes you stronger and more resilient.

5. Find Joy in the Process: Embrace the journey of ancestral eating as an opportunity for growth, exploration, and self-discovery. Discover new foods, flavors, and cooking techniques inspired by ancestral traditions, and find joy in nourishing your body with wholesome, nutrient-dense ingredients. Take pleasure in the simple act of preparing and enjoying meals that support your health and well-being, and let that joy fuel your commitment to ancestral eating.

6. Build a Support System: Surround yourself with a supportive community of like-minded individuals who share your passion for ancestral eating. Whether it's joining online forums, attending local meetups, or connecting with friends and family who support your dietary choices, having a support system can make all the difference on your journey. Share your experiences, seek advice and encouragement from others, and celebrate your successes together.

7. Practice Self-Care: Remember to prioritize self-care as you continue your journey with ancestral eating. Nourish your body, mind, and spirit with plenty of rest, relaxation, and activities that bring you joy and fulfillment. Take time to recharge and rejuvenate, and listen to your body's needs as you navigate the ups and downs of your health and well-being journey.

8. Stay Curious and Open-Minded: Approach your journey with ancestral eating with curiosity and open-mindedness, and be willing to explore new ideas, recipes, and approaches to nutrition. Keep learning and growing, and be open to adjusting your dietary habits based on new information and personal experiences. Stay curious about the impact of ancestral eating on your health and well-being, and let that curiosity drive you to continue exploring and evolving on your journey.

9. Trust the Process: Trust that you are on the right path with ancestral eating, and have faith in the wisdom of your body to guide you towards optimal health and well-being. Trust the process of nourishing your body with whole, unprocessed foods and embracing ancestral eating principles, and have confidence that you are making positive changes that will benefit you in the long run.

10. Be Proud of Yourself: Finally, be proud of yourself for taking ownership of your health and well-being and committing to a journey of self-discovery and growth. Celebrate your courage, determination, and resilience as you continue to prioritize your health and nourish your body with whole, nutrient-dense foods. Be proud of the progress you've made and the positive changes you've experienced, and let that pride inspire you to keep moving forward on your journey with ancestral eating.

In conclusion, remember that your journey with ancestral eating is a personal and transformative one, and you have the power to create the vibrant, healthy life you deserve. Stay committed, stay resilient, and stay true to your health and well-being goals, knowing that every step forward brings you closer to the vibrant, thriving life you envision for yourself. You've got this!

Resources for Further Exploration:

As you continue your journey with ancestral eating, there are many resources available to support and inspire you along the way. Whether you're looking for educational materials, practical guidance, recipe inspiration, or community support, these resources can help deepen your understanding of ancestral eating and empower you to make informed choices for your health and well-being. Here are some valuable resources to explore:

1. **Books**:
"The Paleo Solution" by Robb Wolf
"The Primal Blueprint" by Mark Sisson
"The Paleo Diet" by Loren Cordain
"The Whole30" by Melissa Hartwig Urban and Dallas Hartwig
"Nourishing Traditions" by Sally Fallon Morell

2. Websites and Blogs:
Mark's Daily Apple (marksdailyapple.com)
Robb Wolf (robbwolf.com)
Paleo Leap (paleoleap.com)
Whole30 (whole30.com)
Chris Kresser (chriskresser.com)

3. Podcasts:
The Paleo Solution Podcast with Robb Wolf
The Primal Blueprint Podcast with Mark Sisson
The Balanced Bites Podcast with Diane Sanfilippo and Liz Wolfe
The Chris Kresser Podcast with Chris Kresser
FoundMyFitness Podcast with Dr. Rhonda Patrick

4. Online Communities:
Reddit: r/Paleo, r/Whole30, r/Primal
Facebook Groups: Paleo/Primal Living, Whole30 Community, Ancestral Eating Support Group
Instagram: Follow hashtags such as #ancestraleating, #paleo, #whole30 for inspiration and community support

5. Cooking and Recipe Resources:
Cookbooks focused on ancestral eating, paleo, and Whole30 recipes
Recipe websites such as Nom Nom Paleo, PaleOMG, and The Defined Dish
YouTube channels featuring cooking demonstrations and recipe tutorials for ancestral eating

6. Educational Courses and Workshops:
Online courses on ancestral eating, paleo nutrition, and Whole30 programs
Local workshops and seminars hosted by health and wellness practitioners specializing in ancestral nutrition

7. Health and Wellness Professionals:
Registered dietitians, nutritionists, and health coaches with expertise in ancestral eating
Functional medicine practitioners who incorporate ancestral principles into their practice
Certified Whole30 coaches and mentors who provide personalized guidance and support

8. Scientific Research and Studies:
Explore peer-reviewed scientific journals and publications for research on ancestral eating, paleo nutrition, and related topics
Websites such as PubMed and Google Scholar can help you access scientific studies and literature on ancestral nutrition and its impact on health

9. Documentaries and Films:
"The Paleo Way" (available on DVD and streaming platforms)
"In Search of the Perfect Human Diet" (available on DVD and streaming platforms)
"Fat Fiction" (available on DVD and streaming platforms)

10. Local Resources:
Farmers' markets and local co-ops for sourcing high-quality, locally grown produce, meats, and other ancestral-friendly foods
Community-supported agriculture (CSA) programs for access to fresh, seasonal produce from local farmers
Cooking classes, workshops, and wellness events hosted by local organizations and health practitioners
By exploring these resources and seeking out information and support from trusted sources, you can deepen your knowledge of ancestral eating, discover new recipes and cooking techniques, connect with like-minded individuals, and continue to thrive on your journey towards optimal health and well-being. Remember to approach your exploration with an open mind, stay curious, and embrace the transformative power of ancestral eating as you navigate this exciting journey towards vibrant health and vitality.